HYPERTENSION SECRETS

HYPERTENSION SECRETS

Donald E. Hricik, M.D.

Professor of Medicine
Chief, Division of Nephrology
Case Western Reserve University
    School of Medicine
Medical Director, Transplantation Services
Department of Medicine
University Hospitals of Cleveland
Cleveland, Ohio

Jackson T. Wright, Jr., M.D., Ph.D.

Professor of Medicine
Case Western Reserve University
    School of Medicine
Director of Clinical Hypertension Program
University Hospitals of Cleveland
Chief, Hypertension Section
Louis Stokes Cleveland VAMC
Cleveland, Ohio

Michael C. Smith, M.D.

Professor of Medicine
Division of Nephrology
Case Western Reserve University
School of Medicine
University Hospitals of Cleveland
Cleveland, Ohio

HANLEY & BELFUS, INC./Philadelphia

Publisher: HANLEY & BELFUS, INC.
                Medical Publishers
                210 South 13th Street
                Philadelphia, PA 19107
                (215) 546-7293; 800-962-1892
                FAX (215) 790-9330
                Web site: http://www.hanleyandbelfus.com

Note to the reader: Although the information in this book has been carefully reviewed for correctness of dosage and indications, neither the authors nor the editors nor the publisher can accept any legal responsibility for any errors or omissions that may be made. Neither the publisher nor the editors make any warranty, expressed or implied, with respect to the material contained herein. Before prescribing any drug, the reader must review the manufacturer's current product information (package inserts) for accepted indications, absolute dosage recommendations, and other information pertinent to the safe and effective use of the product described. This is especially important when drugs are given in combination or as an adjunct to other forms of therapy.

Library of Congress Cataloging-in-Publication Data

Hypertension secrets / edited by Donald Hricik, Michael Smith, Jackson Wright.
     p. ; cm.—(The Secrets Series®)
    Includes bibliographical references and index.
    ISBN 1-56053-471-0 (alk. paper)
     1. Hypertension—Examinations, questions, etc. I. Hricik, Donald E. II. Smith,
C. (Michael Charles), 1946- III. Wright, Jackson, 1944- IV. Series.
    [DNLM: 1. Hypertension—Examination Questions. WG 18.2 H9988 2001]
    RC685.H8 H935 2002
    616.1'32'0076—dc21

                                             2001039903

HYPERTENSION SECRETS   ISBN 1-56053-471-0

Last digit is the print number: 9 8 7 6 5 4 3 2 1

DEDICATION

This book is dedicated to our family members: Lynne, Brian, Kevin, Lauren, and Michael Hricik; Lillian, Jackson Sr., Molly, and Adina Wright; Susan, Abigail, Rachel, and Jacob Smith.

CONTENTS

V. THERAPEUTIC PRINCIPLES

CONTRIBUTORS

Hany S. Y. Anton, M.D.
Senior Nephrology and Transplantation Fellow, Case Western Reserve University, University Hospitals of Cleveland, Cleveland, Ohio

David C. Aron, M.D., M.S.
Case Western Reserve University School of Medicine, Cleveland, Ohio

Bruce E. Berger, M.D.
Associate Professor of Medicine, Division of Nephrology, Case Western Reserve University School of Medicine, University Hospitals of Cleveland, Cleveland, Ohio

Ira D. Davis, M.D.
Associate Professor of Pediatrics, Division of Pediatric Nephrology, Department of Pediatrics, Case Western Reserve University School of Medicine; Medical Director of Pediatric Nephrology, Rainbow Babies and Children's Hospital, Cleveland, Ohio

Uday A. Desai, M.D.
Nephrology Fellow, Case Western Reserve University School of Medicine, Cleveland, Ohio

Janice G. Douglas, M.D.
Professor of Medicine and Chief, Division of Hypertension, Case Western Reserve University School of Medicine, University Hospitals of Cleveland, Cleveland, Ohio

Ronald Flauto, D.O.
Nephrology Fellow, Case Western Reserve University School of Medicine, Cleveland, Ohio

Patrick S. T. Hayden, M.D.
Nephrology Fellow, Case Western Reserve University School of Medicine, Cleveland, Ohio

Robert L. Haynie, M.D., Ph.D.
Associate Clinical Professor of Medicine, Associate Dean of Student Affairs, Case Western Reserve University School of Medicine, Huron Road Hospital, Cleveland, Ohio

Donald E. Hricik, M.D.
Professor of Medicine; Chief, Division of Nephrology, Case Western Reserve University School of Medicine; Medical Director, Transplantation Services, Department of Medicine, University Hospitals of Cleveland, Cleveland, Ohio

Arun Kumar, M.D.
Hypertension Fellow, University Hospitals of Cleveland, Cleveland, Ohio

Zuhayr T. Madhun, M.D.
Assistant Professor of Medicine, Case Western Reserve University School of Medicine, Cleveland, Ohio

Lavinia A. Negrea, M.D.
Assistant Professor, Department of Medicine, Case Western Reserve University School of Medicine; Veterans Affairs Medical Center; University Hospitals of Cleveland, Cleveland, Ohio

Andrew S. O'Connor, D.O.
Fellow, Division of Nephrology, Case Western Reserve University School of Medicine, Metro Health Medical Center, Cleveland, Ohio

Kaine C. Onwuzulike
M.D., Ph.D. student, Case Western Reserve University School of Medicine, Cleveland, Ohio

Michael Patterson, D.O.
Nephrology Fellow, Case Western Reserve University School of Medicine, Cleveland, Ohio

Robert Orr, M.D.
Nephrology Fellow, Case Western Reserve University School of Medicine, Cleveland, Ohio

Eleni Pelecanos, M.D., M.P.H.
Assistant Professor of Medicine, Case Western Reserve University School of Medicine, Cleveland, Ohio

Mahboob Rahman, M.D., M.S.
Assistant Professor of Medicine, Divisions of Nephrology and Hypertension, Case Western Reserve University School of Medicine, University Hospitals of Cleveland, Cleveland, Ohio

Michael C. Smith, M.D.
Professor of Medicine, Division of Nephrology, Case Western Reserve University School of Medicine, University Hospitals of Cleveland, Cleveland, Ohio

Beth A. Vogt, M.D.
Assistant Professor, Department of Pediatrics, Case Western Reserve University School of Medicine; Pediatric Nephrologist, Rainbow Babies and Children's Hospital, Cleveland, Ohio

Jackson T. Wright, Jr., M.D., Ph.D.
Professor of Medicine, Case Western Reserve University School of Medicine; Director of Clinical Hypertension, University Hospitals of Cleveland; Chief, Hypertension Section, Louis Stokes Cleveland VAMC, Cleveland, Ohio

PREFACE

Hypertension is a very common disorder, occurring in more than 25% of people living in the United States. Elevations of systemic blood pressure play an important role in the pathogenesis of stroke, heart disease, and end-stage renal disease. Evidence increasingly suggests that control of hypertension can prevent stroke, retard the development and progression of renal failure, reduce left ventricular hypertrophy, and possibly mollify the consequences of coronary artery disease. Although high blood pressure is one of the most common reasons for doctor-office visits, optimal blood pressure control currently is achieved in only 25% of hypertensive patients. The number of pharmacologic agents available to treat hypertension has expanded greatly in the past 20 years, so that safe and effective therapy with one or more drugs should be readily accomplished in most patients. To the extent that hypertension occurs in patients cared for by virtually all medical and surgical specialists, students and house officers should regard basic concepts in the pathophysiology, natural history, and treatment of hypertension as essential elements of training. *Hypertension Secrets* provides information about all aspects of hypertension that should be of value to trainees and to more advanced practitioners who seek a review of essential topics in the field.

Donald E. Hricik, M.D.
Jackson T. Wright, M.D., Ph.D.
Michael C. Smith, M.D.

1. MEASUREMENT OF BLOOD PRESSURE

Arun Kumar, M.D.

1. What is the gold standard method to measure blood pressure (BP)?

Intra-arterial catheterization. This method is not practical in nonhospitalized patients or in an ambulatory setting.

2. List the methods for routine BP measurement in an ambulatory setting.

- Indirect sphygmomanometry (the auscultatory method)
- Oscillometric technique used in home and ambulatory BP monitors
- Ultrasound techniques to measure systolic BP if **Korotkoff sounds** are inaudible or in patients with severe hypotension

3. Who invented sphygmomanometry?

The concept of indirect BP measurement was introduced by Rocci in 1896, when he measured the external pressure necessary to occlude the brachial artery completely to the point when no arterial pulsations were transmitted. The Russian physician **Korotkoff** perfected the method in 1905 and described the auscultatory method and the sounds he used to describe flow through the artery, which are named after him.

4. Describe the principle behind indirect sphygmomanometry.

The artery is occluded by wrapping an inflatable bladder (encased in a nondistensible cuff) around an extremity and inflating the bladder until the pressure in the cuff exceeds the pressure in the artery. When the artery is occluded, the transmitted pulse waves no longer can be palpated or heard distal to the point of occlusion. As the pressure in the bladder is reduced by opening a valve on the inflation bulb, pulsatile blood flow reappears through the partially compressed artery, producing repetitive Korotkoff sounds. The level of the pressure in the inflatable bladder at the appearance of the first Korotkoff sound (reflected by the level on the manometer to which it is connected) is the maximum pressure generated during each cardiac cycle (**systolic pressure**). **Diastolic pressure**, the resting pressure between cardiac contractions, is the level of pressure at which the sounds disappear permanently, indicating that the artery is no longer compressed and blood flow is restored.

5. Describe the standardized requirements for the BP cuff.

Bladder length. The length of the elastic bladder should be sufficient to encircle nearly or completely the patient's arm (at the midpoint between the acromium and olecranon process). As a general rule, the bladder should encircle at least 80% of the arm. A bladder that is too short may not transmit the pressure fully against the artery and result in falsely high readings. For many adults, the standard adult–size bladder (12×23 cm) is not long enough and the large adult–size bladder (15×31–39 cm) is recommended. The thigh-sized bladder (18×36–50 cm) is used in individuals whose arm circumference is 45 to 52 cm and for measuring lower extremity BP. No BP calibration data are available for the thigh cuff.

Bladder width. Bladder width is less important than length but should be at least 40% of the arm circumference.

Bulb and valve. The bulb and valve should be capable of producing a bladder pressure 30 mm Hg above the systolic pressure within 5 seconds of rapid inflation and should hold that pressure until the deflation valve is opened. Deflation should be possible at a rate of 3 mm/sec (or pulse beat). If the pressure cannot be held or smoothly released, the deflation valve is faulty and should be replaced.

6. List cuff sizes recommended by American Heart Association.

PATIENT'S ARM CIRCUMFERENCE	CUFF SIZE TO USE
16–21 cm (6.3–8.2 inches)	Child
22–26 cm (8.6–10.2 inches)	Small adult
27–34 cm (10.6–13.4 inches)	Adult
35–44 cm (13.8–17.3 inches)	Large adult
45–52 cm (17.7–20.5 inches)	Adult thigh

7. Describe the types of sphygmomanometers that are available (see figure, next page).

1. **Mercury.** This is the gold standard for indirect sphygmomanometry. The use of mercury manometers is declining because of concern about mercury toxicity. If used, ensure that the mercury column is at 0 before inflation with a clearly visible meniscus that moves freely when pressure is applied.

2. **Aneroid.** The needle should be at 0 before inflation. The accuracy of the gauge over the entire range of pressures should be checked every 6 months by connecting the aneroid to one limb of a Y-piece; the other limb of the Y-piece is connected to a mercury manometer, and the bottom is connected to a bladder that can be inflated to various levels of pressure. The gauge should be recalibrated if the needle is not at 0 or if the readings differ from the standard mercury manometer by > 4 mm Hg.

3. **Digital/electronic monitors.** These instruments are useful for home BP monitoring and decrease observer bias when used in a clinical setting. Only instruments whose accuracy has been certified by the American Association for the Advancement of Medical Instrumentation (AAMI) or the British Hypertension Society (BHS) should be used. Accuracy may vary between patients, even when using approved instruments. These instruments should be calibrated in each patient against a mercury or recently calibrated aneroid instrument.

8. What extraneous variables may affect BP measurement?
- Food intake and caffeine-containing beverages
- Cigarettes and other tobacco products
- Strenuous exercise within 1 hour of measurement
- Sympathomimetic agents, including eye drops to dilate the pupils
- Full urinary bladder

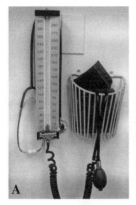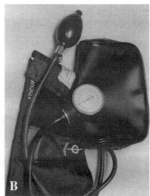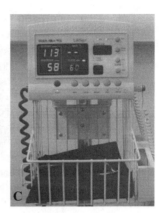

Mercury (*A*), aneroid (*B*), and digital (*C*) sphygmomanometers.

9. Do antihypertensives affect BP measurement?

Yes. If patients are taking antihypertensives, the time since the prior dose should be noted. It is useful to distinguish readings taken at the end of the dosing interval (i.e., 24 hours after a once-a-day dose) from readings taken at or near the time of peak action (i.e., 2–6 hours after ingestion).

10. How does patient position affect measurement of BP?

BP should be measured after 5 minutes of rest, in a quiet relaxed setting, with the legs uncrossed, the feet resting firmly on the floor, not dangling, and the back supported. The practice of measuring BP on the examination table should be avoided because this may elevate BP significantly. Any form of isometric exercise (coughing, Valsalva maneuver) during measurement transiently elevates BP. The subject must be seated comfortably with the midpoint of the upper arm at the level of the heart (approximately the fourth intercostal space) when the subject is seated. The arm should be at the level of the heart when measuring standing and lying BP.

11. What are special instructions for routine BP measurements?

Standing BP and pulse rate should be assessed at every visit in all diabetics, the elderly, and patients on diuretics and sympatholytics (especially α-blockers).

12. Describe in detail the correct technique for measuring BP by auscultation.

1. Palpate the brachial artery and place the cuff so that the midline of the bladder is over the arterial pulsation, then wrap and secure the cuff snugly around the subject's bare upper arm. Avoid rolling up the sleeve in such a manner that it forms a tight tourniquet around the upper arm. Loose application results in overestimation of the pressure. The lower edge of the cuff should be 1 inch (2 cm) above the antecubital fossa, where the head of the stethoscope is to be placed.

2. Inflate the cuff rapidly to 70 mm Hg, and increase by 10-mm Hg increments while palpating the radial pulse. Note the level of pressure at which the pulse disappears and subsequently reappears during deflation. This procedure, the palpatory method, provides a preliminary approximation of the systolic BP. The palpatory

method is particularly useful to avoid underinflation of the cuff in patients with an auscultatory gap and discomfort from overinflation in patients with low BP.

3. Switch the stethoscope head to low frequency (bell), and place it over the brachial artery pulsation. This should be above and medial to the antecubital fossa but below the lower edge of the cuff. Hold it firmly in place, ensuring that the head makes contact with the skin around its entire circumference. Wedging the head of the stethoscope under the edge of the cuff may free up one hand but results in considerable extraneous noise.

4. Inflate the bladder rapidly and steadily to a pressure 20 to 30 mm Hg above the level previously determined by palpation, then partially unscrew the valve and deflate the bladder pressure at a rate of approximately 2 mm Hg per pulse beat, while listening for the appearance and disappearance of the Korotkoff sounds.

5. As the pressure in the bladder falls, note the level of the pressure on the manometer at the first appearance of repetitive sounds (**phase 1**) and at the muffling of these sounds (**phase 4**) and when they disappear (**phase 5**).

6. After the last Korotkoff sound is heard, the cuff should be deflated slowly for another 10 mm Hg, to ensure that no further sounds are audible. The **systolic (phase 1)** and **diastolic (phase 5)** pressures should be recorded immediately, rounded off (upward) to the nearest 2 mm Hg. In children and when sounds are heard nearly to a level of 0 mm Hg, the phase 4 pressure also should be recorded.

7. The measurement should be repeated after at least 30 seconds and the two readings averaged.

8. In the initial evaluation of a hypertensive patient, BP should be measured in both arms and in the legs. BP should be measured in younger individuals with suspicion of coarctation.

13. Summarize the steps for systolic and diastolic BP pressure measurements.
- Estimate systolic BP by palpation
- Place stethoscope gently over point of maximal pulsation of brachial artery
- Inflate cuff to 30 mm Hg above estimated systolic pressure
- Reduce pressure at rate of 2 to 3 mm Hg per second
- Take reading of systolic pressure when repetitive, clear tapping sounds appear for two consecutive beats
- Take reading of diastolic pressure when repetitive sounds disappear

BIBLIOGRAPHY

1. Joint National Committee on Prevention, Detection, Evaluation, and Treatment of High Blood Pressure: The Sixth Report of the Joint National Committee on Prevention, Detection, Evaluation, and Treatment of High Blood Pressure. Arch Intern Med 157:2413–2446, 1997.
2. Perloff D, Grim C, Flack J, et al: Human blood pressure determination by sphygmomanometry. Circulation 88:2460–2462, 1993.
3. Petrie JC, O'Brien ET, Littler WA, de Swiet M: Recommendations on blood pressure measurement. BMJ 293:611–615, 1986.
4. Recommendations for routine blood pressure measurement by indirect cuff sphygmomanometry. American Society of Hypertension. Am J Hypertens 5:207–209, 1992.

2. CLINICAL EVALUATION OF HYPERTENSION

Arun Kumar, M.D.

1. List the objectives of clinical evaluation of a patient with hypertension.

1. To identify potentially correctable causes of the elevated blood pressure (BP)

2. To identify other cardiovascular risk factors or concomitant disorders that may influence prognosis and guide treatment

3. To assess end-organ damage (especially that which may affect therapy) and establish baseline abnormalities

4. To assess previous treatment experience and obstacles to therapy

2. What are the questions to be asked in a medical history?

- Known duration and levels of elevated BP
- Family history of hypertension and its sequelae
- Symptoms suggesting secondary hypertension
  - Paroxysmal headache, palpitations, flushing, weight loss, sweating (**pheochromocytoma**; see Chapter 11)
  - Muscle weakness (**hypokalemia** and **primary aldosteronism**; see Chapter 10)
  - Weight loss or gain, heat intolerance, change in stamina (**hypothyroidism or hyperthyroidism**; see Chapter 13)
  - Sleep disturbance, snoring, daytime somnolence (**sleep apnea sydromes**; see Chapter 13)
- Patient history or symptoms of target organ damage, such as angina, heart and kidney failure, history of stroke or transient ischemic attack, claudication, and sexual dysfunction
- Cardiovascular risk factors, including diabetes mellitus, smoking history, dyslipidemia, and family history of early atherosclerotic disease (age < 55 in male and < 65 in female first-degree relatives)
- History of recent changes in weight, leisure time physical activity, and cigarette or other smoking use
- Dietary assessment, including intake of salt, alcohol, and calories
- History of all prescribed and over-the-counter medications, including herbal remedies, and illicit drugs, some of which may raise BP or interfere with the effectiveness of antihypertensive drugs (see Chapter 13)
- Results and adverse effects of previous antihypertensive therapy (adverse reactions, including sexual dysfunction)
- Psychosocial and environmental factors (e.g., family situation, employment status and working conditions, educational level) that may influence adherence to treatment

3. List symptoms or signs suggesting secondary hypertension.

Headaches, tremor, palpitations, perspiration, pallor, tachycardia, weight loss (**pheochromocytoma** or **hyperthyroidism**)

Obesity, increased facial hair, truncal distribution of fat (**hyperadrenalism**)

Skin lesions (striae in **hyperadrenalism** and oral and facial neuromas and café au lait spots suggesting **multiple endocrine hyperplasia type 3**)

Muscle weakness or cramps (**primary aldosteronism**)

Holosystolic epigastric bruit or bruit with diastolic component in the periumbilical area or flanks (**renovascular disease**)

Radial-femoral pulse delay (**coarctation of aorta**)

4. What are the findings to look for on physical examination in a hypertensive patient?

- Two or more BP measurements separated by 2 minutes with the patient either supine or seated and after standing for at least 2 minutes
- Verification in the contralateral arm (if values differ by > 4 mm Hg, the values in the arm with the highest readings should be used)
- Measurement of height, weight, and waist circumference
- Funduscopic: Hypertensive retinopathy graded as per Keith-Wagener classification:
  Grade 1: Thickening, irregularity, and tortuosity of arterioles
  Grade 2: Above plus constriction of retinal veins at arterial crossings (arteriovenous nicking)
  Grade 3: Above plus flame-shaped hemorrhages or cotton wool exudates (or both)
  Grade 4: Above plus papilledema
- Neck: Carotid bruits, distended veins, thyroid (nodule suggesting medullary carcinoma of thyroid and **pheochromocytoma [multiple endocrine hyperplasia type 2]** and goiter suggesting **hypothyroidism**)
- Lungs: Rales (**congestive heart failure**) and bronchospasm, which would limit consideration of β-blockers
- Heart: Abnormalities in rate and rhythm, increased size, precordial heave, murmurs (especially aortic insufficiency and isolated systolic hypertension), and gallops
- Abdomen: Bruits (especially a diastolic component), enlarged kidneys (**polycystic kidney disease**), masses, and abnormal aortic pulsation
- Extremities: Diminished or absent peripheral arterial pulsations, bruits, and edema; assessment for pseudohypertension (Osler's maneuver)
- Neurologic assessment: To establish baseline physical findings

5. What is pseudohypertension?

Pseudohypertension is thought to occur in elderly persons who have rigid arteries. The indirect sphygmomanometer can overestimate the true intra-arterial pressure because increased pressure is required for the cuff to compress a stiff artery. Pseudohypertension should be suspected in elderly patients with relatively high BP but no evidence of target-organ damage.

6. Define Osler's maneuver.

A palpable radial or brachial artery after the BP cuff has been inflated above the peak systolic pressure. Although this physical finding is compatible with pseudohypertension, some clinicians argue that the maneuver is not specific or sensitive enough to rule out true hypertension.

7. What laboratory and diagnostic tests should be performed as part of the evaluation of hypertension?

Routine laboratory tests recommended before initiating therapy to determine:
- The presence of **target organ damage:** Serum creatinine, electrocardiogram, and urinalysis for protein and cells
- **Cardiovascular risk factors:** Fasting glucose, total and high-density lipoprotein cholesterol

Additional tests to consider:
- Microalbuminuria or timed urinary protein collection
- Blood calcium, uric acid, fasting lipid profile, glycosylated hemoglobin, thyroid-stimulating hormone
- Echocardiography to determine the presence of left ventricular hypertrophy

8. Which patients require additional diagnostic testing?

Patients
1. Whose age, history, examination, severity of hypertension, or initial laboratory findings suggest secondary causes
2. With resistant hypertension defined by BP > 140/90 mm Hg (160/90 mm Hg for patients > 60 years old) on maximal doses of at least three appropriate antihypertensives
3. With previous good BP control who show acute unexplained exacerbation
4. With hypertension associated with grade 3 or 4 retinopathy
5. With new-onset hypertension after age 60
6. With suspected new or worsening target organ damage

BIBLIOGRAPHY

1. Joint National Committee on Prevention, Detection, Evaluation, and Treatment of High Blood Pressure: The sixth report of the Joint National Committee on Prevention, Detection, Evaluation, and Treatment of High Blood Pressure. Arch Intern Med 157:2413–2446, 1997.

3. ARTIFACTUAL HYPERTENSION AND AMBULATORY BLOOD PRESSURE MONITORING

Arun Kumar, M.D.

1. What is artifactual hypertension?

The conventional clinic measurement of blood pressure (BP) does not reflect actual intravascular BP, resulting in the incorrect classification of a normotensive patient as a hypertensive patient. This situation could be due to factors involving the physician, the patient, or both.

2. List the sources for error in underestimating or overestimating BP.

Cuff size
Arm position
Observer errors
White-coat hypertension
Rate of cuff inflation and deflation
Auscultatory gap
Technical sources

3. Discuss cuff size and arm position and how they influence BP measurement.

Cuff Size

The size of the cuff relative to the diameter of the arm is crucial. The most common mistake is to use a cuff that is too small, resulting in overestimation of BP. The appropriate cuff size is one in which the bladder width is 40% of the circumference of the midpoint of the upper arm, and the length of the bladder is 80% of the circumference of the arm.

Arm Position

There is a progressive increase in BP of about 4 to 5 mm Hg when the arm is moved from the horizontal to vertical position. To avoid measurement error associated with arm position, BP always should be measured with the arm supported at the level of the heart.

4. What kinds of observer errors are common?

Errors resulting from diminished auditory acuity
Errors resulting from observer digit preference—a disproportionate number of readings ending in certain digits, especially 0

5. Define white-coat hypertension.

BP taken by physicians can be significantly higher than pressures taken by the patient at home using the same technique and maintaining the same posture. Pressures often are higher when taken by physicians compared with nurses or technicians. Twenty-four-hour ambulatory BP monitoring or multiple clinic readings at multiple visits are required when white-coat hypertension is a consideration.

6. How do cuff inflation and deflation affect BP measurement?

The rate of inflation has little effect on BP, but a slow deflation rate (<2 mm Hg/sec) can overestimate diastolic BP. The general rule is that the deflation rate should be at the rate of 2 to 3 mm Hg/sec.

7. Define the auscultatory gap.

The loss and appearance of the **Korotkoff sounds** that occur during cuff deflation between systolic and diastolic pressures, in the absence of cardiac arrhythmias. If the presence of the auscultatory gap is not recognized, spuriously high diastolic pressures or low systolic pressures are recorded; this is avoided by measuring systolic BP by the palpatory method before measuring by the auscultatory method. Auscultatory gap is most often seen in patients with severe arteriosclerosis. It is a sign of **target organ damage**.

8. List technical sources of error.

1. The position of the mercury column should be at the level of the heart.

2. Mercury in the column should read 0 when no pressure is applied and should fall freely during deflation.

3. Aneroid meters should be checked against a mercury manometer at 0 pressures and when pressure is applied to the cuff. If the needle is not at 0 or if the difference in pressure between the aneroid and mercury manometers is >4 mm Hg, the meter requires recalibration.

CONTROVERSY

9. Discuss the role of ambulatory BP monitoring.

In general, monitoring BPs outside of the hospital or clinic environment has been performed increasingly either as:

- Self-monitoring with a home sphygmomanometer or
- Continuous monitoring with an automated device over an extended period of time

Ambulatory BP monitoring can provide multiple readings during different times of day and may assist the physician in decision making. It is generally believed that home readings avoid the pressor response that typifies **white-coat hypertension**.

Most studies published to date have shown ambulatory BP readings to be superior to office readings in predicting **target organ involvement**, such as left ventricular hypertrophy.

Despite these trends and advantages, routine ambulatory BP monitoring has not been recommended by the sixth report of the Joint National Committee, based in part on the argument that, in most clinical trials, treatment of BP and outcomes of treatment have been based on office (not home) readings. Data indicate that patients with slightly elevated BPs in the office setting but with normal home readings tend to have elevated peripheral vascular resistance, insulin resistance, and other metabolic abnormalities that put them at risk for sustained hypertension and cardiovascular disease.

BIBLIOGRAPHY

1. Joint National Committee on Prevention, Detection, Evaluation, and Treatment of High Blood Pressure: The sixth report on prevention, detection, evaluation, and treatment of high blood pressure. Arch Intern Med 157:2413–2446, 1997.
2. Julius S, Mejia A, Jones K, et al: "White coat" verusus "sustained" borderline hypertension in Tecumseh, Michigan. Hypertension 16:617–623, 1990.
3. Mansoor GA, White WB: Ambulatory blood pressure is a useful clinical tool in nephrology. Am J Kidney Dis 30:591–605, 1997.

4. HYPERTENSIVE CRISES

Bruce E. Berger, M.D.

1. What is a hypertensive crisis?

A syndrome of acute severe hypertension that, at the time of presentation, is associated either with end-organ damage (referred to as a **hypertensive emergency**) or with no end-organ damage (a **hypertensive urgency**).

2. When are the terms *malignant hypertension* and *accelerated hypertension* used to describe severe hypertension?

Traditionally, these two terms were used to describe an acute increase in blood pressure (BP) in an individual with preexisting hypertension. The distinction between the two terms was made by funduscopic examination. **Malignant hypertension** denotes the presence of papilledema (**Keith-Wagener grade IV retinal changes**), whereas **accelerated hypertension** denotes the presence of hemorrhages, cotton-wool spots, and hard exudates and no papilledema (**Keith-Wagener grade III retinopathy**). Given the interobserver variability in detecting papilledema (if not the fading art of performing funduscopy) and the identical clinical approach and management of the two conditions, the distinction between them is increasingly moot. To a certain extent, malignant hypertension and accelerated hypertension have been supplanted by and fit within the category of **hypertensive emergencies**.

3. What is the clinical significance of preexisting hypertension in hypertensive emergencies?

In the setting of underlying, chronic, and sustained hypertension that precedes the accelerated phase, autoregulation of blood flow has occurred to a higher baseline BP. Acute end-organ damage generally occurs at BPs higher than those seen in individuals in whom there was no preexisting hypertension (e.g., the preeclamptic/eclamptic pregnant woman or cocaine user).

4. Define severe chronic hypertension.

The presence of severe hypertension that is associated with chronic end-organ changes, such as hypertensive nephrosclerosis or cardiomyopathy. In the absence of a history of chronic hypertension and end-organ damage, however, it can be otherwise indistinguishable from a hypertensive urgency.

5. What BP values define the severe hypertension that is present in a hypertensive crisis?

There is no absolute value. Conventionally, a diastolic BP of ≥120 mm Hg is used. The range for diastolic BPs is 100 to 180 mm Hg and for systolic BPs is 150 to 290 mm Hg. Because of the implications regarding end-organ damage and therapy, it is important to assess accurately the context of the clinical presentation for each patient.

6. Give examples that differentiate chronic hypertension from a hypertensive emergency.

1. An otherwise asymptomatic 28-year-old black man presents to the emergency department after a motor vehicle accident. He is found to have a BP of 210/124 mm Hg. Funduscopy reveals no papilledema, hemorrhages, or exudates. There is no S3 gallop or volume overload. The electrocardiogram reveals left ventricular hypertrophy, and the creatinine level is 1.8 mg/dL. This patient most likely has **severe chronic hypertension**.

2. A 28-year-old white woman with an otherwise normal pregnancy presents at 32 weeks' gestation with a several-hour history of confusion, nausea, and vomiting. In the emergency department, she is found to have a BP of 160/104 mm Hg and proteinuria. She has a **hypertensive emergency**.

7. Given the range of BPs associated with hypertensive crises, what determines the urgency of treatment?

The most critical factor in determining the urgency of treatment is the recognition of an acute deterioration of a **vital end-organ function** (i.e., **hypertensive emergency**). In this setting, BP is generally best lowered over several minutes to the limit to reverse end-organ damage.

When the severe hypertension is believed to be acute but without symptoms or signs (i.e., **hypertensive urgency**), the BP is lowered over several hours to prevent the evolution to a hypertensive emergency.

When the severe hypertension is believed to be **chronic** (with or without end-organ sequelae), the BP is generally lowered within several days (see Chapter 22).

8. Describe what triggers a hypertensive crisis.

Among all the causes associated with a hypertensive crisis, the common thread is an abrupt increase in **systemic vascular resistance**. In many settings, the increased vasoconstriction occurs because of enhanced activity of the renin-angiotensin system or enhanced release of norepinephrine. As a result, tissue ischemia ensues, and this stimulates further the release of renin or catecholamines, such as norepinephrine. The critical concern in this vicious cycle is the development of vascular damage. When endothelial injury occurs, unfolding and potentially devastating outcomes include the following:

1. Impaired autoregulation of organ perfusion (e.g., acute renal failure, acute myocardial infarction, pulmonary edema) from acute fibrinoid necrosis

2. Microangiopathic hemolytic anemia

3. Local activation of the coagulation system

Depending on whether preexisting hypertension has been present, the media of smooth muscle cells have proliferated (**onion skinning**) because of increased local production of cytokines and growth factors potentiating even more tissue hypoperfusion. Further contributions to this deteriorating picture appear to be related, in some instances at least, to the presence of increased levels of vasopressin, endothelin, and cortisol.

9. List the underlying causes associated with hypertensive crises.
Essential hypertension
Secondary hypertension

Coarctation of the aorta
Renovascular (e.g., renal artery stenosis, fibromuscular dysplasia, arteritis, embolism)
Renoparenchymal
    Primary (e.g., glomerulonephritis)
    Secondary (e.g., scleroderma crisis, systemic lupus erythematosus, hemolytic uremic syndrome, vasculitis)
    Endocrine (e.g., pheochromocytoma, primary mineralocorticoid excess states [rare])
Eclampsia/preeclampsia
Sympathomimetic stimulation
    Cocaine
    Amphetamine
    Acute clonidine withdrawal
    Acute β-blocker withdrawal
    Monoamine oxidase inhibitor interactions
Cerebrovascular
    Head trauma
    Infarction
    Hemorrhage
    Tumors

10. What are the clinical presentations of a hypertensive emergency?

The varied clinical presentations reflect the end-organ manifestations of the abrupt and severe elevation in BP and include
• Cerebrovascular
• Cardiovascular
• Renal
• Microangiopathic hemolytic anemia

The severity of the hypertension is not the sole determinant of clinical expression. In patients with acute hypertensive emergency without preexisting hypertension, their vessel walls lack the protective effects of myointimal proliferation seen in patients with chronic hypertension. The clinical expression of acute end-organ failing is present at lower BPs.

11. Describe a cerebrovascular presentation of a hypertensive emergency.

Symptoms suggestive of neurologic dysfunction are observed frequently, with approximately 60% of patients complaining of **headaches** and approximately 25% complaining of dizziness. **Hypertensive encephalopathy**, which in addition would include nausea and vomiting, impaired cognitive function (confusion, somnolence, delirium, coma), or seizures, is less common. Although present in the initial reports of malignant hypertension in 60% of patients, visual complaints now are less common. Focal neurologic findings suggest a transient or localized lesion from thrombosis, a cerebral hemorrhage, or a subarachnoid hemorrhage.

12. Describe a cardiovascular presentation of a hypertensive emergency.

Congestive heart failure and **pulmonary edema** are present in approximately

10% of patients. Features of **ischemic heart disease** (angina in approximately 4% and myocardial infarction in approximately 4%) are common. Aortic dissection is present in <1% of patients. Patients with underlying ischemic heart disease have a significant risk of renovascular disease (approximately 20%). **Flash pulmonary edema** is common in this setting and is often transient and self-limited.

13. Describe a renal presentation of a hypertensive emergency.

The frequent presence of **azotemia** (approximately 30%) is a reflection of the underlying renal parenchymal process responsible for the hypertensive crisis (e.g., a **rapidly progressive glomerulonephritis**), the presence of underlying chronic hypertension (i.e., hypertensive nephrosclerosis), the presence of acute damage from fibrinoid necrosis, or a combination of these conditions. The arterial findings of fibrinoid necrosis resolve within 3 weeks of controlled BP. As with cerebrovascular disease, the preexisting status of the autoregulatory curve and the extent of insult to the autoregulatory process determine the degree and duration of acute renal failure. The influence of these factors on the autoregulation of renal blood flow is illustrated in the figure. Hypokalemia is observed commonly on presentation and reflects stimulation of the renin-angiotensin-aldosterone system.

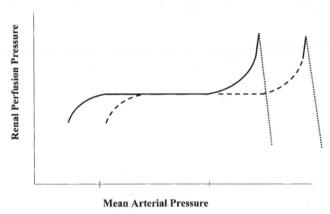

Mean Arterial Pressure

Solid line represents normotensive autoregulatory curve.Dashed line represents the autoregulatory curve in chronic hypertension.

14. Describe the presentation of microangiopathic hemolytic anemia.

The presence of thrombotic microangiopathy usually is associated with and probably potentiates the severity of renal failure. This may reflect the concomitant presence of thrombocytopenia, increased fibrin degradation products and fibrinogen, and intravascular coagulation and their effects on damaged endothelium.

BIBLIOGRAPHY

1. Healton EB, Brust JC, Feinfeld DA, Thomson GE: Hypertensive encephalopathy and the neurologic manifestations of malignant hypertension. Neurology 32:127–132, 1982.
2. Kitiyakara C, Guzman NJ: Malignant hypertension and hypertensive emergencies. J Am Soc Nephrol 9:133–142, 1998.
3. Murphy C: Hypertensive emergencies. Emerg Med Clin North Am 13:973–1007, 1995.

5. EPIDEMIOLOGY OF HYPERTENSION

Jackson T. Wright, Jr., M.D., Ph.D.

1. What is the prevalence of hypertension in the United States?
- More than 40 million of the noninstitutionalized and nonmilitary population (> 50 million overall) or almost ¼ of the U.S. population have a blood pressure > 140/90 or report taking antihypertensives (see Table).
- Hypertension prevalence increases with increasing age.
- The prevalence has been decreasing over the last 3 decades (see Figure).
- African Americans have the highest prevalence of hypertension (> 40% higher than U.S. whites).
- Mexican Americans have a lower prevalence than U.S. whites but also have one of the lowest rates of satisfactory blood pressure control.

Prevalence of Hypertension, by Race and Sex, Age 18 and Older

	AGE-ADJUSTED PERCENT	UNADJUSTED PERCENT	ESTIMATED POPULATION[†] (IN THOUSANDS)
Overall*	24.2	24.0	43,186
Male*	25.9	24.7	21,287
Female*	22.2	23.4	21,900
Black, non-Hispanic	32.4	28.4	5,672
White, non-Hispanic	23.3	24.6	34,697
Mexican American	22.6	14.3	1,143

*Includes all racial groups
† Estimate from unadjusted percent
Adapted from Burt VL, Whelton P, Roccella EJ, et al: Prevalence of hypertension in the US adult population: Results from the Third National Health and Nutrition Examination Survey, 1988–1991. Hypertension 25:305–313, 1995.

2. What are the clinical consequences of hypertension?
The clinical consequences are predominantly vascular; cerebrovascular, coronary artery, peripheral vascular, renal vascular damage, and retinopathy. In addition, the increased cardiac workload may result in left ventricular hypertrophy leading to an increased rate of both diastolic and systolic dysfunction (and congestive heart failure).

Hypertensive patients have twice the risk of myocardial infarction, a threefold risk of stroke and peripheral vascular disease, and an approximately fourfold increased risk of heart failure. In addition, hypertension is the second leading cause of end-stage renal disease in the U.S. (See figure, top of next page.)

3. Describe the profile of blood pressure elevation associated with hypertension.
- Both diastolic blood pressure (DBP) and systolic blood pressure (SBP) increase until about age 55. At about that time, SBP and DBP begin to diverge with SBP continuing to increase whereas DBP begins to decline (see Chapter 20).

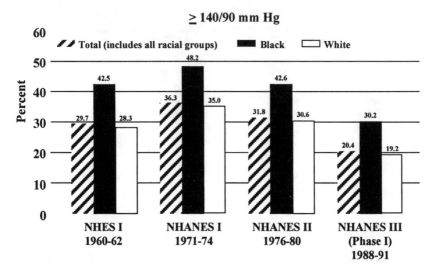

Trends in the age-adjusted prevalence of hypertension by race in patients aged 18–74 years. (Adapted from Burt VL, Whelton P, Roccella EJ, et al: Prevalence of hypertension in the US adult population: Results from the Third National Health and Nutrition Examination Survey, 1988–1991. Hypertension 25:305–313, 1995.)

- In addition to its association with increased age, the increase in the difference between SBP and DBP (pulse pressure) is associated with cardiovascular risk factors and a powerful predictor of future cardiovascular events.
- Isolated systolic hypertension is the most common form of hypertension, and about 65% of people with hypertension over the age of 65 have isolated systolic hypertension.
- Hypertension severity is more frequently defined by DBP before age 40, by either or both DBP and SBP between age 40 and 60 years, and by SBP after age 60.
- After age 60, over 94% of cases of hypertension will be accurately classified as stage 1–3 by knowing only the SBP whereas only 18% will be accurately defined by the DBP.

4. What is the relative clinical significance of pulse pressure, SBP, and DBP?

Hypertension-related morbidity and mortality correspond best with pulse pressure, followed closely by SBP, then DBP. Although pulse pressure is a more accurate predictor of cardiovascular disease (CVD) risk, SBP is simpler to use and nearly as accurate. DBP correlates with CVD risk through young adulthood. However, after age 50, for any given SBP, DBP is inversely associated with CVD risk (the lower the DBP, the higher the risk of CVD). (See figure, top of next page).

5. What effect do other risk factors have on patients with hypertension?

The majority of hypertensive patients have one or more concomitant risk factors (e.g., hypercholesterolemia (35%), diabetes mellitus (35%), cigarette use). The adverse CVD risk of hypertension is magnified by the presence of other risk factors

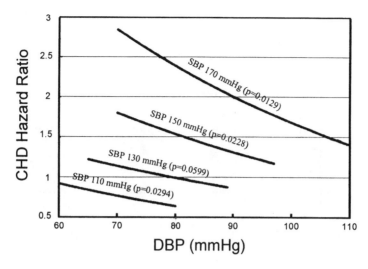

Relationship of congestive heart disease (CHD) to diastolic blood pressure (DBP) and systolic blood pressure (SBP). (From Franklin SS, Khan SA, Wong ND, et al: Is pulse pressure useful in predicting risk for coronary heart disease? The Framingham Heart Study. Circulation 100:353, 1999, with permission.)

and requires a more aggressive approach to all risk factors. Thus, CVD risk can increase from twofold in those with hypertension as the only risk factor to more than 20-fold higher risk in hypertensive patients with diabetes, hypercholesterolemia, cigarette use, and left ventricular hypertrophy.

BIBLIOGRAPHY

1. Burt VL, Whelton P, Roccella EJ, et al: Prevalence of hypertension in the US adult population: Results from the Third National Health and Nutrition Examination Survey, 1988–1991. Hypertension 5:305–313, 1995.
2. Franklin SS, Khan SA, Wong ND, et al: Is pulse pressure useful in predicting risk for coronary heart disease? The Framingham Heart Study. Circulation 100:354–360, 1999.
3. Joint National Committee: The sixth report of the Joint National Committee on Prevention, Detection, Evaluation, and Treatment of High Blood Pressure (JNC-VI). Bethesda, MD, US Department of Health and Human Services, National Heart, Lung, and Blood Institute, 1997, NIH publication no. 98-4080.
4. Kannel WB: Some lessons in cardiovascular epidemiology from Framingham. Am J Cardiol 37:269–282, 1976.

6. PATHOPHYSIOLOGY OF ESSENTIAL (PRIMARY) HYPERTENSION

Janice G. Douglas, M.D., and Kaine C. Onwuzulike

1. What hemodynamic mechanisms contribute to the presence of essential hypertension?

Blood pressure is the product of cardiac output and peripheral vascular resistance. A variety of factors influence cardiac output and vascular resistance (see tables) and, therefore, contribute to blood pressure regulation. Although the exact mechanisms of essential hypertension have not yet been elucidated, several variables have been suggested to contribute to sustained blood pressure elevations in humans, as discussed in the following questions.

Mediators of Peripheral Vascular Resistance

INCREASE RESISTANCE	DECREASE RESISTANCE
Angiotensin II	Bradykinin
Norepinephrine	Nitric oxide
Epinephrine	Atrial natriuretic peptide
Vasopressin (ADH)	Prostaglandins
Endothelin	Prostacyclins
Eicosanoids: thromboxane A_2	

Mediators of Cardiac Output

INCREASED CARDIAC OUTPUT	DECREASED CARDIAC OUTPUT
Aldosterone/mineralcorticoids	Hemorrhage
Vasopressin	Loss of salt and water
Increased intravascular volume	Decreased intravascular volume
Increased sympathetic nervous system activity	

2. What humoral mechanisms play a role in the pathophysiology of essential hypertension?

The renin-angiotensin system (RAS) plays a pivotal role in the regulation of blood pressure and is a key mediator of target organ damage, cardiovascular events, and progression of renal disease. RAS regulates both peripheral vascular resistance directly through the effects of angiotensin II (AII) and intravascular volume indirectly through the actions of both AII and aldosterone. Many humoral mediators, both autocrine and paracrine, influence peripheral vascular resistance and contribute to the modulation of blood pressure. Other players in the humoral milieu of blood pressure regulation include endothelin, a potent vasoconstrictor, vasopressin (antidiuretic hormone/[ADH]), and the natriuretic peptides.

3. What is the renin-angiotensin system, and how does it influence blood pressure?

The classic RAS consists of renin produced by the kidneys, renin substrate (angiotensinogen) produced by the liver, and angiotensin-converting enzyme (ACE) localized primarily in the lungs (and to a minor degree in the vasculature), and AII, which delivers the end-organ effects most notable for this system (see figure). The biological effects of the RAS system are widespread and long lasting; however, the rapid actions of this system are a concerted effort to support the circulation when it is threatened by intravascular volume depletion.

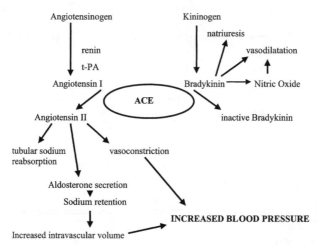

4. How are renin levels altered in hypertensive individuals?

Renin levels, which are typically elevated during states of volume depletion and decreased in states of volume excess, are below normal in 30% of hypertensive patients, normal in 60%, and above normal in the remainder of hypertensive individuals. Even "normal" levels of renin and AII are inappropriate in hypertensive individuals.

5. What are the angiotensin receptor subtypes, locations, and end-organ effects?

Multiple receptor subtypes for AII have been described (e.g., AT_1, AT_2, AT_4). However, virtually all of the characterized actions of AII are mediated by the AT_1 receptor, which is a member of the superfamily of peptide hormone receptors, with seven membrane-spanning domains coupled to G-proteins. The AT_1 receptor is found throughout the vasculature and many other organ systems. The AT_2 receptor is much more prevalent during fetal life.

Actions of Angiotensin II that Influence Blood Pressure Regulation

LOCATION	AT_1	AT_2
Arterial smooth muscle	Vasoconstriction, proliferation	Not present in vasculature
Adrenal gland	Aldosterone secretion, cortisol and catecholamine release	Inhibition of aldosterone release
Sympathetic nervous system	Catecholamine release	?
Kidney	Tubular sodium reabsorption, increased vascular resistance	Natriuresis
Vascular endothelium	Endothelin production	
Myocardium	Increased contractility, ventricular hypertrophy	Dilation of coronary endothelium

6. How does insulin influence the development and progression of hypertension?
In many patients with hypertension, especially those with type II diabetes, there is altered insulin-dependent transport of glucose into peripheral tissues ("insulin resistance") that leads to a state of hyperinsulinemia—a major risk factor for the development of hypertension and cardiovascular disease. A number of well-documented studies have shown an association between insulin resistance and hypertension. In fact, hypertension is twice as common in type II diabetics as in the general population. It is generally accepted that these disorders are interrelated etiologically; however, the precise mechanisms have not been validated.

7. What is syndrome X, and how does it affect hypertension and cardiovascular risk?
Syndrome X is a compilation of cardiovascular risk factors that include:
- Impaired glucose tolerance (hyperinsulinemia)
- Type II diabetes mellitus
- Obesity
- Low HDL cholesterol
- Elevated triglyceride
- Elevated free fatty acids
- Hypertension
- Left ventricular hypertrophy
- Increased platelet aggregation
- Enhanced sympathetic nerve activity
- Accelerated atherosclerotic disease

Syndrome X is associated with a two- to threefold increase in rates of cardiovascular morbidity and mortality.

8. How does hyperinsulinemia cause or exacerbate the progression of hypertension?
- Insulin has been shown to stimulate renal sodium retention, resulting in increased intravascular volume.
- Insulin increases sympathetic nervous system activity, leading to increased peripheral resistance and cardiac output.
- Insulin has a mitogenic effect on smooth muscle cells, leading to vascular smooth muscle proliferation that can facilitate atherogenesis and decreased arterial compliance
- Insulin can lead to altered cell membrane transport resulting in increased intracellular calcium. This increase leads to increased vascular resistance.

9. What is the relationship between insulin resistance and essential hypertension?
More than 50% of patients with essential hypertension exhibit evidence of insulin resistance. This is probably related to the high prevalence of obesity among patients with essential hypertension and the fact that insulin resistance is associated with obesity.

10. What are the sites of origin and actions of the natriuretic peptides?
Atrial natriuretic peptide (ANP) is synthesized primarily in the right atrium of the heart and released in response to increased distention of the right atrium associated with increased intravascular volume. Brain natriuretic peptide (BNP) is synthesized and stored in the central nervous system and atrial cells. C-type natriuretic peptide (CNP) is produced by the endothelium. As their names imply, all of the natriuretic peptides promote natriuresis and lowering of blood pressure. Equally

important actions include the inhibition of renin and aldosterone release. Furthermore, ANP and CNP have antimitogenic properties.

11. What is the association between endothelin and hypertension and cardiovascular disease?

Endothelin, produced by the endothelial cells of the vasculature, exhibits vasconstrictive properties in the coronary bed and mixed vasodilatory and vasoconstrictive properties in the peripheral vasculature. Endothelin also induces cardiac myocyte hypertrophy. Endogenous endothelin levels are often elevated in patients with essential hypertension, but the causality of this relationship has yet to be determined.

12. Describe vasopressin and its role in the regulation of intravascular volume and blood pressure regulation.

Vasopressin (antidiuretic hormone) is a nonapeptide released from the posterior pituitary gland in response to reduced intravascular volume or blood pressure. It is one of the most potent circulating vasoactive substances.

13. What is neuropeptide Y?

Neuropeptide Y, a 36-amino-acid peptide, has been implicated as a contributor to the regulation of blood pressure. It is found extensively throughout the central and peripheral nervous systems in neurovascular junctions and acts as a direct vasoconstrictor, simultaneously potentiating the effects of norepinephrine (NE) and AII.

14. What is the relationship between vasopressin and essential hypertension?

Plasma concentrations of vasopressin have been found to be elevated in up to 30% of males with hypertension. Vasopressin levels in blood also have been shown to correlate directly with systolic and diastolic pressures in hypertensive males.

15. Are there racial differences in plasma vasopressin levels? If so, what are their implications in essential hypertension?

Plasma vasopressin levels have been reported to be higher in blacks than in whites. Selective inhibition of vasopressin V_1 receptors has been shown to lower mean arterial blood pressure in blacks (~28 mm Hg) but not whites.

16. What roles do the brain stem, hypothalamus, and cortical centers play in the pathophysiology of hypertension?

Lesions of the nucleus solitarius have been associated with increased sympathetic activity and can lead to fulminant hypertension in animal models. The paraventricular nucleus has a well-established role in arterial pressure regulation due to its production of ADH, which promotes water retention through its actions on the renal collecting ducts.

17. What role does the sympathetic nervous system play in the initiation and maintenance of essential hypertension?

A widely accepted hypothesis suggests that the sympathetic nervous system is a critical initiating factor in the development of essential hypertension in humans but has little if any effect on maintaining chronically elevated blood pressure. This hypothesis suggests that hypertension begins as a syndrome of high cardiac output caused by overactivity of cardiac sympathetic nerves. This "hyperdynamic" phase eventually leads to sustained heightened systemic vascular resistance, which is the hallmark of essential hypertension. During this period of chronically elevated arterial pressure, structural changes such as vascular hypertrophy are believed to contribute to the maintenance of increased vascular resistance.

An alternate and less popular view, yet one that appears to be more consistent with clinical observations to date, is that the sympathetic nervous system not only is the initiating factor in the development of essential hypertension, but also directly contributes to maintenance of elevated arterial pressure. This view suggests that the sympathetic nervous system creates a dynamic and morbid mix of high cardiac output and chronically elevated systemic vascular resistance.

18. What evidence is there for sympathetic nervous system overactivity in both the early and established phases of chronic hypertension?

Several well-conducted studies demonstrate inappropriate sympathetic nervous system activity in all phases of human hypertension. Norepinepherine is the major catecholamine agonist acting on the peripheral α- and β-adrenergic receptors, and norepinephrine levels have been noted to be higher in patients with essential hypertension than in the general population. It is generally accepted that in, the early phases of hypertension, sympathetic nervous system overactivity exists as evidenced by elevated plasma concentrations of norepinephrine, increased muscle sympathetic nerve traffic, and increased plasma renin (the downstream mediator angiotensin II). Increased norepinephrine stimulates renin release from the kidneys via the β-adrenergic receptor system (see figure).

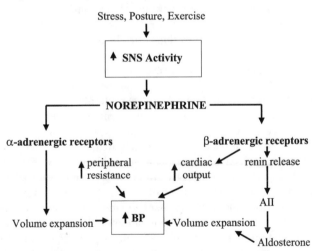

In established hypertension, the normal to elevated plasma levels of norepinepherine in the setting of increase arterial pressure are actually inappropriate because plasma norepinepherine should be physiologically suppressed when arterial pressures are elevated. Further evidence of excessive sympathetic nervous system activity in established hypertension comes by way of organ specific radiotracer spillover studies in which markedly elevated cardiac and renal sympathetic activity is observed in essential hypertension. These influences are thought to sustain an inappropriately high level of high cardiac output, increased preload, increased contractility of the heart, and increased peripheral vascular resistance.

19. How are endothelial dysfunction and vascular hyperreactivity linked to the pathophysiology of essential hypertension?
Nitric oxide (NO) is the most potent physiologic arterial dilator known. Endothelium-dependent vasodilatation, mediated by NO, has been found to be abnormal in forearm and coronary resistance vessels of patients with essential hypertension. Vasodilator responses have also been shown to be blunted in patients with hypertension and their normotensive offspring. The elevated and sustained sheer stress concomitant with high blood pressure leads to the endothelial dysfunction seen in long-standing hypertension.

20. What role do intracellular calcium $[Ca^{2+}]_i$ and magnesium $[Mg^{2+}]_i$ play in the determination of blood pressure?
Elevated $[Ca^{2+}]_i$ and/or suppressed $[Mg^{2+}]_i$ levels have been found in patients with essential hypertension, obesity, and type II diabetes mellitus. Higher $[Ca^{2+}]_i$ and lower $[Mg^{2+}]_i$ are associated with elevated blood pressure, increased cardiac hypertrophy, increased vascular resistance, hyperinsulinemia, and insulin resistance.

21. What is the role of intracellular sodium $[Na^+]_i$ in hypertension? Describe the variations of intracellular sodium concentrations found in black and non-black populations.
Average intracellular sodium concentrations are consistently higher in African Americans as compared to whites. A positive correlation between intracellular sodium levels and hypertension prevalence has been established in that increased $[Na^+]_i$ leads to increased Na^+/Ca^{2+} exchange activity, which ultimately increases intracellular calcium leading to increased vascular tone.

22. Describe salt sensitivity and its role in the pathophysiology of hypertension.
Dietary sodium can have heterogeneous effects in hypertensive individuals. Salt-sensitive hypertension is a form of essential hypertension defined by an increment in mean arterial blood pressure ≥ 10 mmHg with a salt challenge. By contrast, salt-resistant individuals have negligible changes in blood pressure associated with a salt challenge. It appears that almost two thirds of hypertensive African Americans are salt-sensitive compared to less than half of non–African American patients with hypertension. The distinction of being characterized as salt-sensitive carries important clinical and therapeutic considerations in that it allows for behavior modification to be used (in conjunction with pharmacologic therapy) as an effective early mechanism for blood pressure control. It has been observed that social groups that typically ingest < 50–100 mEq/day of sodium have a substantially lower incidence of both hypertension and cardiovascular disease than groups in whom habitual sodium intake is greater. In addition to the greater prevalence of salt sensitivity in African Americans and the elderly, recent data have shown that salt sensitivity in normotensive individuals is associated with a significantly greater age-related increase

in blood pressure than in salt-resistant subjects, implying that the age-related rise in blood pressure may be a reflection of salt-sensitivity. Some investigators have suggested that stress-related increments in sympathetic nervous system activity and accompanying sodium and water retention underlie salt sensitivity.

23. What populations are more susceptible to salt sensitivity of blood pressure regulation?
- African Americans
- Elderly
- Diabetics
- Individuals with insulin resistance

24. What is the estimated prevalence of salt sensitivity in the general population?
It is estimated that up to two thirds of blacks and up to one third of whites are salt sensitive.

25. What are the characteristics of nonmodulator hypertension?
Nonmodulator hypertension refers to salt-sensitive hypertensive patients, with pathophysiologically normal or elevated plasma renin activity, who exhibit abnormal aldosterone responses in the face of volume manipulation. Nonmodulator hypertensive patients differ in their renal hemodynamic responses to salt-challenged and -deprived states. There appears to be a very strong familial predisposition in nonmodulation.

26. How does the morbidity and mortality of hypertension in blacks compare to nonblack populations?
The prevalence of hypertension in blacks is among the highest in the world. In black adults 20 years and older, the prevalence is estimated to be 34% in men, and 31% in women; this is contrasted with 24% for the overall US population. Hypertension develops earlier in life and is of a greater magnitude in blacks than in whites. The earlier onset, higher prevalence, and greater incidence of severe hypertension in blacks contributes to an 80% higher mortality rate from stroke, a 50% higher mortality rate from heart disease, and over a 300% greater incidence of end-stage renal disease compared to the general population.

27. Describe the main pathophysiologic and hemodynamic properties of hypertension that are unique to the African-American population.
- Lower plasma renin activity
- Decreased renal perfusion with heightened renal vascular resistance
- Increased peripheral vascular resistance
- Increased incidence of nephrosclerosis
- Greater rate of hyperinsulinemia
- Decreased urinary kallikrein excretion
- Decreased prostaglandin E_2 (potent vasodilator) activity
- Decreased ANP activity
- Increased levels of endothelin-1

28. How does the plasma renin activity of blacks compare with nonblack populations?

Blacks typically exhibit a more volume-dependent, salt-sensitive form of hypertension than whites, and usually have lower basal and stimulated levels of plasma renin activity. Low plasma renin levels are generally associated with plasma volume expansion.

29. Can the blood pressure variation observed in the general population be explained by genetic factors?

Many believe that environmental influences are far more important than genetic determinants in the development of essential hypertension. Approximately 30–50% of the blood pressure variation observed in the general population can be explained by genetic factors, with the remainder left to environmental and social influences such as socioeconomic status and diet.

BIBLIOGRAPHY

1. Bakris G, Burszten M, Gavras I, et al: Role of vasopressin in essential hypertension: Racial differences. J Hypertens 15:545–550, 1997.
2. Dzau VJ, Burt DW, Pratt RE: Molecular biology of the renin-angiotensin system. Am J Physiol 255:F563–F573, 1988.
3. Ferro CJ, Webb DJ: Endothelial dysfunction and hypertension. Drugs 53(suppl 1):30–41, 1997.
4. Goodfriend TL, Elliott ME, Catt KJ: Angiotensin receptors and their antagonists. N Engl J Med 334:1649–1654, 1996.
5. Insel PA: Adrenergic receptors: Evolving concepts and clinical applications. N Engl J Med 334:580–585, 1996.
6. Linz W, Wiemer G, Gohlke P, et al: Contributions of kinins to the cardiovascular actions of angiotensin-converting enzyme inhibitors. Pharmcol Rev 47:25–49, 1995.
7. Michel MC, Rascher W: neuropeptide Y: A possible role in hypertension. J Hypertens 13:385–395, 1995.
8. Nasjletti A, Arthur C: The role of eicosanoids in angiotensin-dependent hypertension. Hypertension 31:194–200, 1997.
9. Wilkins MR, Redondo J, Brown LA: The natriuretic-peptide family. Lancet 349:1307–1310, 1997.

7. NATURAL HISTORY OF HYPERTENSION

Jackson T. Wright, Jr., M.D., Ph.D.

1. What are the major consequences of hypertension?

- Accelerated athero-arteriosclerosis causing coronary artery disease, ischemic stroke, ischemic nephropathy, peripheral artery disease, and retinopathy
- Hemodynamic complications of congestive heart failure, hemorrhagic stroke, aortic dissection, and encephalopathy
- Death

2. How does blood pressure vary with age?

In the industrialized world, blood pressure increases with increasing age. In response to decreased arterial compliance, the pulse pressure widens as systolic blood pressure increases and diastolic blood pressure decreases with aging (see Chapter 20). Untreated, about 1% of hypertensives will progress to malignant hypertension. Blood pressure is extremely variable with greatest variability noted in:

Diabetics and others with autonomic dysfunction
The elderly
Hypertensive patients
Obese patients

3. What is the typical clinical course of hypertension?

- Unless there is a secondary cause, hypertension usually has a long progressive clinical course (see Table).
- The clinical course can be highly variable depending on genetic and environmental exposures and patient variables.
- Each stage allows opportunities for intervention to modify the clinical course.
- Throughout most of its history, hypertension has few symptoms. Symptoms are principally related to the target organ damage rather than to the elevated blood pressure.

Time Course of Hypertension

AGE	STAGE OF CLINICAL COURSE	POTENTIAL INTERVENTION
Birth	Genetic-prenatal	Prenatal care, ? genetic intervention
Birth–30 yrs	Risk factor evolution	Primary prevention
20–40 yrs	Hypertension subclinical TOD	Primary prevention, early treatment
30–50 yrs	Established hypertension with evolving TOD	Aggressive treatment risk factor intervention
> 40 yrs	Clinical events/mortality	Premortality secondary prevention

TOD = target organ damage.

4. What factors identified in hypertensives are associated with an increased risk of complications?
- Age and duration of blood pressure elevation
- Blood pressure level

    40% of patients in the first VA Cooperative Trial with DBP between 115 and 129 mmHg developed severe complications over an average follow-up of 16 months.

    55% of participants in this trial with DBP between 90 and 114 mmHg (mean = 157/101) developed a morbid event.
- Presence of clinical target organ damage—left ventricular hypertrophy (LVH), renal insufficiency, ischemic changes on electrocardiogram (ECG)
- Diabetes (doubles the cardiovascular event rate after adjusting for other risks)
- Socioeconomic status
- ? African-American ethnicity

5. Name some clinical signs of progressive hypertension.
- Early markers

    Retinopathy (arteriolar narrowing)

    S_4 gallop

    Echocardiographic evidence of increased left ventricular mass
- Established hypertension

    Retinopathy (retinal artery-venous [A-V] nicking)

    More pronounced S_4

    Clear evidence of LVH on echocardiogram and increased voltage on ECG (*note:* electrocardiographic assessment of ventricular hypertrophy has very high false positive rate in African Americans)

    Decreased glomerular filtration rate

    Microalbuminuria
- Established target organ damage

    Increased heart size,

    Precordial heave

    Retinopathy (A-V nicking with tortuousity)

    Bruits of large arteries

    Vessels sclerotic by palpation

    LVH criteria on ECG with ST-T changes

    Increased serum creatinine
- Clinical events (e.g., myocardial infarction, stroke) or mortality

BIBLIOGRAPHY

1. Joint National Committee: The Sixth Report of the Joint National Committee on Prevention, Detection, Evaluation, and Treatment of High Blood Pressure (JNC-VI). Bethesda, MD, US Department of Health and Human Services, National Heart, Lung, and Blood Institute, 1997, NIH publication no. 98-4080.
2. Kaplan NM: Primary hypertension: Natural history. In Kaplan NM: Clinical Hypertension, 5th ed. Baltimore, Williams & Wilkins, 1990, pp 112–135.

8. RENAL PARENCHYMAL HYPERTENSION

Michael C. Smith, M.D.

1. Why is hypertension important in patients with renal disease?

1. Hypertension associated with renal parenchymal disease is the most common form of **secondary hypertension**; 5% of all hypertensive patients have underlying renal disease.

2. Hypertension is prevalent in renal disease. Of patients with pre–end-stage renal disease (ESRD), > 80% are hypertensive, and hypertension is present in 90% by the time ESRD ensues.

3. In addition to increasing cardiovascular morbidity and mortality, hypertension in patients with renal disease accelerates the loss of renal function. **Glomerular filtration rate** (GFR) declines more rapidly in hypertensive patients with renal disease compared with their normotensive counterparts.

2. How does renal disease cause hypertension?

The kidney plays a central role in blood pressure (BP) regulation because of its ability to regulate salt excretion. A positive **salt balance** is crucial to the initiation and maintenance of renal parenchymal hypertension. Activation of the intrarenal renin-angiotensin-aldosterone system (RAAS) and increased central sympathetic outflow have been linked to the development of hypertension in pre-ESRD and ESRD.

3. What evidence supports a crucial role for salt in the initiation and maintenance of renal parenchymal hypertension?

1. Many studies have shown that hypertensive subjects with mild-to-moderate renal impairment have increased total body sodium. Small changes in total body sodium often precede frank elevations of BP or increments in serum creatinine.

2. Increases in dietary salt expand extracellular fluid volume and augment arterial pressure in most patients with renal dysfunction. This hypertensive effect of dietary salt loading is inversely related to GFR and most evident in patients with ESRD.

3. Dietary salt restriction or diuretic administration in patients with pre-ESRD or salt removal during dialysis in patients with ESRD decreases total body sodium, extracellular fluid volume, and BP in renal parenchymal hypertension.

4. What data indicate an important role for the RAAS in renal parenchymal hypertension?

Activation of the RAAS increases BP not only through the vasoconstrictor action of angiotensin II (AII), but also because of augmented renal sodium reabsorption mediated by AII and aldosterone. In many, but not all, patients with pre-ESRD, plasma renin activity (PRA) and AII concentration are increased and correlate with BP. AII receptor blockade in some hypertensive patients with renal parenchymal disease results in a decrement in BP that is inversely proportional to baseline PRA.

In 10% to 20% of patients with ESRD, BP is clearly renin dependent. In these patients, PRA often is increased, and BP does not normalize with salt removal during dialysis. Before the advent of minoxidil and angiotensin-converting enzyme (ACE) inhibitors, bilateral nephrectomy often was required to control BP in ESRD patients with resistant hypertension and elevated PRA.

5. How does increased sympathetic nervous system activity contribute to hypertension in renal disease?

Many studies have shown increased plasma norepinephrine concentrations in hypertensive patients with pre-ESRD. This enhanced sympathetic nervous system activity not only directly increases BP by increasing **cardiac output** and **total peripheral resistance**, but also indirectly augments BP by stimulation of the **RAAS**. Activation of renal sympathetic nerves increases sodium reabsorption, contributing to volume expansion and further increments in BP. The reason that patients with renal disease exhibited enhanced sympathetic nervous system activity had been unclear. Emerging experimental and clinical data support the concept that in diseased kidneys there is increased renal afferent sympathetic nerve traffic, which signals the anterior hypothalamus to increase central sympathetic outflow.

6. How are prostaglandins (PGs) involved in renal parenchymal hypertension?

Renal and extrarenal PGs play important roles in regulating **vascular tone** and **salt excretion**. Some PGs ($PGF_{2\alpha}$ and thromboxane A_2) are vasoconstrictor and antinatriuretic, whereas others (PGE_2 and PGI_2) are vasodilator and natriuretic. On

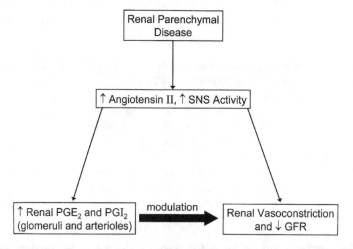

Renal parenchymal disease is often associated with augmented production of angiotensin II and increased activity of the sympathetic nervous system (SNS). The effect is twofold: first, a direct intrarenal vasoconstrictor effect that decreases renal blood flow (RBF) and GFR, and second, an increased synthesis of vasodilators and natriuretic prostaglandins (PG). The latter modulates intrarenal vasoconstriction. Inhibition of intrarenal PG production by nonsteroidal anti-inflammatory drugs results in unopposed intrarenal vasoconstriction with a further decline in RBF and GFR. (From Smith MC, Rahman M, Dunn MJ: Hypertension associated with renal parenchymal disease. In Schrier RW, Gottschalk CW (eds): Diseases of The Kidney. Philadelphia, Lippincott, Williams & Wilkins, 2001, in press; with permission).

balance, however, stimulation of endogenous PG synthesis tends to decrease BP. A decrease in renal PG production theoretically could contribute to renal parenchymal hypertension. PG production tends to be normal or increased in hypertensive patients with renal disease, however. This is due to the fact that AII and enhanced sympathetic nervous system activity directly stimulate renal synthesis of PGE_2 and PGI_2 (see figure), and they modulate the direct intrarenal vasoconstrictor and antinatriuretic effects of AII and the SNS.

This has important therapeutic implications. Inhibition of renal PG production by administration of nonsteroidal anti-inflammatory drugs (NSAIDs) to hypertensive patients with renal disease can decrease salt excretion and exacerbate hypertension as well as causing acute-on-chronic renal failure. Sulindac and piroxicam may be more renal sparing than other nonselective cyclooxygenase (COX) inhibitors. Selective COX-2 inhibitors have the same adverse intrarenal hemodynamic profile as their nonselective counterparts. All NSAIDs should be used cautiously, if at all, in hypertensive patients with renal disease and only with careful monitoring of renal function and serum potassium.

7. Describe the effect hypertension has on renal function in patients with renal disease.

Hypertension accelerates the decline of renal function. This effect is mediated largely by hemodynamic mechanisms. The figure shows a schematic representation of glomeruli from a normal individual and a patient with hypertension and renal disease.

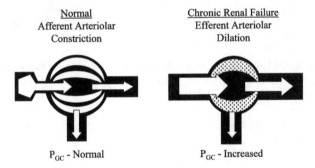

Intrarenal respone to systemic hypertension.

Under normal circumstances (*left panel*), renal blood flow (RBF) and GFR are held constant over a wide range of mean arterial pressures (MAP) by constriction or dilation of the afferent arteriole. If systemic BP increases, the afferent arteriole constricts and intraglomerular capillary pressure (P_{GC}) remains normal. In renal disease (*right panel*), enhanced PG synthesis dilates the afferent arteriole and results in transmission of systemic BP to the glomerulus with a consequent increase in P_{GC}. This elevated glomerular pressure results in further hydraulically mediated damage, proteinuria, glomerulosclerosis, and a more rapid decrease in GFR.

8. Summarize the pathophysiologic mechanisms responsible for the accelerated decline in renal function in renal parenchymal hypertension.

See figure, top of next page.

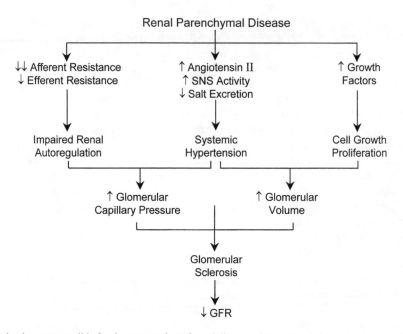

Mechanisms responsible for the progression of renal disease when systemic hypertension coexists with renal parenchymal disease. GFR = glomerular filtration rate; SNS = sympathetic nervous system. (From Smith MC, Dunn MJ: Hypertension in renal parenchymal disease. In Laragh JH, Brenner BM (eds): Hypertension: Pathophysiology, Diagnosis, and Management. New York, Raven Press, 1995, p 2094, with permission.)

9. Does treatment of hypertension slow the progression of kidney disease?

Absolutely. Reduction of BP ameliorates the progression of diabetic and non-diabetic renal disease primarily by decreasing P_{GC}.

10. What should be the goal BP in hypertensive patients with pre-ESRD?

In general, 130/80 mm Hg.

In patients with moderate-to-heavy proteinuria (1–3 g/24 h or > 3 g/24 h), ≤ 125/75 mm Hg.

11. Describe the initial therapeutic strategy in treating renal parenchymal hypertension.

Because salt retention is central to the pathogenesis of hypertension in renal disease, a logical initial therapeutic approach requires dietary sodium restriction to 80 to 100 mmol/d. When **dietary salt restriction** is in place, most patients still require **diuretic therapy** to achieve desired salt balance. Thiazide diuretics are generally ineffective with creatinine clearances < 30 mL/min. Hypertensive patients with this degree of renal insufficiency require loop-blocking diuretics, generally in a twice-a-day dosing regimen to achieve the requisite natriuresis. Diuretic therapy should be increased until the patient is free of edema. This approach can normalize BP in 25% to 30% of patients; the remainder require additional drug therapy to achieve goal BP.

12. If diuretic therapy does not control BP, what drug classes should be added next?

In patients with pre-ESRD, an antihypertensive drug should be logical from a pathophysiologic perspective, have a favorable side-effect profile, exert a beneficial effect in cardiovascular morbidity and mortality, and retard the progression of renal disease.

1. **ACE inhibitors** and **angiotensin receptor blockers (ARBs)** exert a unique renoprotective effect independent of their ability to lower BP. These drugs should be added to dietary salt restriction and diuretic therapy if BP is not at goal, provided that no contraindication (i.e., hyperkalemia, angioedema) exists.

2. **Calcium channel antagonists** reduce BP despite extremes of dietary salt intake and are a logical next step if further reduction of BP is required.

3. **Centrally acting sympatholytics** are excellent drugs from a pathophysiologic and practical point and often control BP in patients who have been resistant to the first three drug classes.

13. Is it the norm to require three or more drug classes in patients with renal parenchymal hypertension to achieve goal BP?

Yes, especially if the goal is $\leq 125/75$ mm Hg.

14. Are there risks to the use of ACE inhibitors or ARBs in hypertensive patients with renal insufficiency?

Yes. Two are most important.

1. **Hyperkalemia** can occur and is more likely with more severe renal dysfunction and in the face of additional constraints on potassium homeostasis (e.g., diabetes, nonselective β-blockade, digitalis). Serum potassium should be monitored frequently.

2. ACE inhibition or AII blockade can result in **acute-on-chronic renal failure.** These drugs dilate the efferent arteriole and in the face of a dilated afferent arteriole make GFR exquisitely dependent on systemic BP. If BP decreases excessively, filtration is compromised, and acute-on-chronic renal failure ensues (i.e., *no BP, no pee pee*).

15. What is the approach to the treatment of hypertension in patients with ESRD?

Of hypertensive patients on maintenance hemodialysis, 80% to 90% become normotensive if sufficient salt and water are removed by dialysis to achieve a true dry weight. The remaining patients require nondiuretic antihypertensive therapy. Because the pathogenesis of hypertension in hemodialysis patients is similar to that in patients with pre-ESRD, selection of pharmacologic agents should be comparable: ACE inhibitors, ARBs, calcium channel antagonists, and centrally acting sympatholytics are logical and effective selections.

BIBLIOGRAPHY

1. Converse RL, Jacobsen TN, Toto RP, et al: Sympathetic overactivity in patients with chronic renal failure. N Engl J Med 327:1912–1918, 1992.
2. GISEN Group: Randomized placebo-controlled trial of effect of ramipril on decline in glomerular filtration rate and risk of terminal renal failure in proteinuric nondiabetic nephropathy. Lancet 349:1857–1863, 1997.

3. Ihle BU, Whitworth JA, Shahinfar S, et al: Angiotensin-converting enzyme inhibition in nondiabetic renal insufficiency: A controlled double-blind trial. Am J Kidney Dis 27:489–495, 1996.
4. Lewis EJ, Hunsicker LG, Bain RP, Rohde KD: The effect of angiotensin-converting enzyme inhibition on progression of diabetic nephropathy. N Engl J Med 329:1456–1462, 1993.
5. Ligtenberg G, Blankestijn PJ, Oey PL, et al: Reduction of sympathetic hyperactivity by enalapril in patients with chronic renal failure. N Engl J Med 340:1321–1328, 1999.
6. Kshirsagar AV, Joy MS, Hogan SL, et al: Effect of ACE inhibitors in diabetic and nondiabetic chronic renal disease: A systematic overview of randomized placebo-controlled trials. Am J Kidney Dis 35:695–707, 2000.
7. Maschio G, Alberti D, Janin G, et al: The effect of the angiotensin-converting enzyme inhibitor benazepril on the progression of chronic renal insufficiency. N Engl J Med 334:939–945, 1996.
8. Peterson JC, Adler S, Burkhart JM, et al: Blood pressure control, proteinuria, and the progression of renal disease: The modification of diet in renal disease study. Ann Intern Med 123:754–762, 1995.
9. Rahman M, Smith MC: Chronic renal insufficiency: A diagnostic and therapeutic approach. Arch Intern Med 158:1743–1752, 1998.
10. Schlondorff D: Renal complications of nonsteroidal anti-inflammatory drugs. Kidney Int 44:643–653, 1993.
11. Smith MC, Dunn MJ: Role of the kidney in blood pressure regulation. In Jacobson HR, Striker GE, Klahr S (eds): The Principles and Practice of Nephrology. Philadelphia, B.C. Decker, 1995, pp 362–370.

9. RENOVASCULAR HYPERTENSION

Robert Orr, M.D., and Donald E. Hricik, M.D.

1. What is renovascular hypertension?

High blood pressure (BP) caused by occlusive disease of one or both main renal arteries or their branches. The presence of renovascular hypertension can be confirmed only by showing that high BP is improved or cured after correction of the occlusion.

2. Discuss the pathophysiology of renovascular hypertension.

Renovascular hypertension results from activation of the renin-angiotensin-aldosterone axis mediated by ischemia. Decreased perfusion to the affected kidney results in the release of renin, which accelerates the conversion of angiotensinogen to angiotensin I. Angiotensin-converting enzyme (ACE) converts angiotensin I to angiotensin II, a peptide with potent vasoconstrictor properties. Angiotensin II also stimulates the adrenal gland to release aldosterone, leading to renal sodium retention.

The pathophysiology of renovascular hypertension varies depending on whether renal occlusive disease occurs in one kidney in a patient with two kidneys and a normal contralateral kidney versus a solitary kidney in a patient with no contralateral kidney or in bilateral renal artery stenosis in a patient with two kidneys. Using language derived from animal models, these two circumstances sometimes are referred to as the **two-kidney, one-clip model** and the **one-kidney, one-clip model**. In the two-kidney model, the ischemic kidney secretes renin and retains salt and water, but the normal contralateral kidney exhibits a pressure natriuresis that leads to negative sodium balance, further exacerbating the release of renin. In the one-kidney model, absence of a contralateral kidney prevents sodium loss. Extracellular volume expansion ensues, plasma renin activity is suppressed, and hypertension persists largely because of volume overload.

3. List the causes of renovascular hypertension.

Common (approximately 95% of cases)	Rare (approximately 5% of cases)
• Atherosclerosis	• Neurofibromatosis
• Fibromuscular dysplasia	• Extrinsic compression
	• Congenital anomalies
	• Radiation fibrosis
	• Arterial thromboembolism
	• Vasculitis

4. Define fibromuscular dysplasia.

A nonarteriosclerotic occlusive vascular disease of unknown cause. The disorder occurs most commonly in young or middle-aged women and is uncommon in African-Americans. The dysplastic process primarily involves the renal arteries, but other vascular beds (e.g., carotid and cerebral vessels) can be involved. Four pathologic variants have been described. **Medial fibroplasia** is the most common (accounting for 70% of all cases) and is recognized angiographically by the classic **string of beads** appearance (see figure). The less common variants are intimal, perimedial, and adventitial fibrous dysplasia. Fibromuscular dysplasia most often involves the middle-to-distal two thirds of the renal artery.

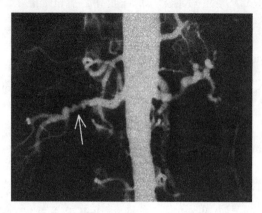

Renal angiogram demonstrating medial fibrous dysplasia in a main renal artery. (From Hricik DE: Renovascular hypertension. In Hricik DE, Sedor JR, Ganz MB (eds): Nephrology Secrets. Philadelphia, Hanley & Belfus, 1999, p 194, with permission.)

5. List clinical characteristics that are typical of patients with renovascular hypertension.

1. Progression in the severity of chronic hypertension
2. Recent onset of hypertension
3. Malignant hypertension
4. Moderate hypertension in a patient with diffuse vascular disease (especially if the patient is a smoker)
5. Early (age <25 years) or late (age >60 years) onset
6. Renal failure during treatment with an ACE inhibitor or angiotensin receptor blocker
7. Abdominal or flank bruit
8. Recurrent episodes of flash pulmonary edema

6. What is the gold standard test to make a diagnosis of renovascular hypertension?

Angiography. Digital subtraction angiography is preferred in some centers in an effort to minimize the amount of administered contrast dye. Digital studies may not provide adequate images of the peripheral branches of the arterial tree, however. Angiographic techniques can detect anatomic abnormalities, but they do not provide information about the functional significance of a renal artery stenosis. Most clinicians agree, however, that luminal narrowing of ≥70% is usually clinically significant.

7. List other noninvasive tests that have been used to screen for renovascular disease.

Duplex ultrasonography	ACE inhibitor–stimulated renography
Magnetic resonance angiography	ACE inhibitor–stimulated peripheral
Spiral CT scan	renin activity

8. What are the limitations of duplex ultrasonography in the diagnosis of renovascular hypertension?
1. The main renal artery is not visualized in 25% of cases.
2. Small accessory renal arteries often are not detected.
3. The procedure is highly operator-dependent.

9. Are anatomic renovascular lesions always associated with hypertension?
No. Many studies have shown that in normotensive patients undergoing nonrenal angiography (e.g., cardiac catheterization or angiography of the peripheral vasculature), renovascular lesions are detected in >30% of patients.

10. How do angiotensin inhibitors cause renal failure in patients with renovascular disease?
ACE inhibitor–induced renal failure first was described in patients with bilateral renal artery stenosis or renal artery stenosis involving a solitary kidney. Under circumstances in which the entire renal mass is hypoperfused as a consequence of arterial occlusion, intrarenal hemodynamics are altered such that autoregulation of glomerular filtration rate (GFR) becomes critically dependent on the effects of angiotensin II on the efferent (postglomerular) capillaries. When angiotensin II is inhibited by an ACE inhibitor (or by an angiotensin receptor blocker), postglomerular resistance decreases. In theory, renal blood flow is maintained or increased, but GFR may fall dramatically. The hemodynamic pattern is described best as a dissociation in the autoregulation of renal blood flow and GFR.

11. How does ACE inhibitor renography diagnose renovascular disease?
GFR is estimated by the clearance of a radioisotope under baseline conditions and again after administration of an ACE inhibitor. A decrease in the GFR after ACE inhibitor administration suggests the presence of a functionally significant occlusion.

12. What are the objectives of therapy in patients with renovascular disease?
1. Control systemic BP
2. Preserve renal function

13. List the available treatments for patients with renovascular hypertension.
Medical therapy (antihypertensive drugs)
Percutaneous transluminal angioplasty (with or without stenting)
Surgery

14. Discuss the management principles underlying the choice of therapy for patients with renovascular hypertension.
The choice of therapy depends on the severity of the systemic hypertension, pathologic process (i.e., atherosclerosis versus fibromuscular dysplasia), presence or absence of renal impairment, location of the lesion, and presence of comorbid conditions (e.g., coronary or cerebrovascular disease) that may affect life expectancy.

Medical therapy may control BP adequately but is not likely to decrease the risk of progressive renal impairment resulting from renal ischemia. Medical therapy may contribute to progressive ischemic injury by reducing systemic pressure and further reducing perfusion to the affected kidney.

For patients who are candidates for invasive therapy, **percutaneous transluminal angioplasty** is preferred because it can be performed without general anesthesia or prolonged hospitalization. The main limitations of angioplasty are technical failures, vascular accidents (e.g., dissection or rupture), and recurrence of stenoses. Angioplasty is the treatment of choice for patients with **fibromuscular dysplasia**.

15. Name the surgical techniques employed to treat renovascular hypertension.

Aortorenal bypass with autogenous hypogastric artery or saphenous vein

Aortorenal bypass graft

Renal endarterectomy

Splenorenal bypass (in patients with severe aortic disease on the left side)

Hepatorenal bypass (in patients with severe aortic disease on the right side)

16. List the indications for medical therapy in patients with renovascular hypertension.

1. Patients with bilateral or segmental lesions deemed to be nondilatable and inoperable

2. Patients with high operative risks (e.g., elderly patients with concomitant coronary or cerebrovascular disease)

3. Patients who refuse invasive therapy

17. How does the location of an atherosclerotic renal artery stenosis influence therapy?

Angioplasty is technically difficult to perform in atherosclerotic lesions in the proximal portion of the renal artery, especially if the lesion involves the renal ostium. Such lesions tend to recur with great frequency. Bypass surgery is preferred in such cases if the patient is an operative candidate. Angioplasty is more successful in the management of atherosclerotic lesions involving the distal two thirds of the main renal artery.

18. Can renal artery stenosis result in proteinuria?

Yes. Occasionally, patients with renal artery stenosis present with frank nephrotic syndrome. Proteinuria in such cases probably results from the effects of high levels of angiotensin on glomerular permeability to macromolecules. The presence of heavy proteinuria does not rule in the presence of parenchymal renal disease or rule out renal artery stenosis. In patients with renovascular hypertension, heavy proteinuria may remit completely after successful revascularization.

19. List the indications for surgery in patients with renovascular hypertension.

1. Ostial or near-ostial atherosclerotic lesions (usually treated with a bypass graft)

2. Occlusive lesions in distal branches of the renal arterial tree (may require bench surgery or nephrectomy)

3. Progressive fibrous dysplastic lesions not responsive to angioplasty (usually occurring in patients with adventitial or intimal variants)

4. Progressive hypertension or renal failure despite transient improvements with angioplasty

CONTROVERSY

20. How common is renovascular hypertension?
The prevalence of renovascular hypertension varies widely depending on the population being studied and the type of tests performed to make the diagnosis. Autopsy studies suggest that 40% of adults have at least mild narrowing of the renal arteries, but many cases may be clinically insignificant. Among severely hypertensive patients referred to tertiary care centers, the prevalence of renovascular hypertension may be >20% in patients studied with angiography. Most authorities agree, however, that renovascular disease probably accounts for high BP in 5% of the general population of patients with hypertension.

BIBLIOGRAPHY

1. Davidson RA, Wilcox CS: Newer tests for the diagnosis of renovascular disease. JAMA 268:3353–3358, 1992.
2. Hricik DE, Dunn MJ: Angiotensin-converting enzyme inhibitor-induced renal failure: Causes, consequences, and diagnostic uses. J Am Soc Nephrol 1:845–858, 1990.
3. Mann SJ, Pickering TG: Detection of renovascular hypertension: State of the art, 1992. Ann Intern Med 117:845–853, 1992.
4. Martinez-Maldonado M: Pathophysiology of renovascular hypertension. Hypertension 17:707–719, 1991.
5. Olin JW, Piedmonte MR, Young JR, et al: The utility of duplex ultrasound scanning of the renal arteries for diagnosing significant renal artery stenosis. Ann Intern Med 122:833–838, 1995.
6. Plouin PF, Darne B, Chantellier G, et al: Restenosis after a first percutaneous transluminal angioplasty. Hypertension 21:89–96, 1993.
7. Rimmer JM, Gennari FJ: Atherosclerotic renovascular disease and progressive renal failure. Ann Intern Med 118:712–719, 1993.
8. Ying CY, Tift CP, Gavras H, Chobanian AV: Renal revascularization in the azotemic hypertensive patient resistant to therapy. N Engl J Med 311:1070–1075, 1984.

10. HYPERALDOSTERONISM

Zuhayr T. Madhun, M.D., and David C. Aron, M.D., M.S.

1. Define primary hyperaldosteronism.

A syndrome characterized by excessive production of aldosterone leading to sodium retention, weight gain, and hypertension, usually accompanied by hypokalemia and metabolic alkalosis.

2. Describe the different causes of primary hyperaldosteronism.

The most common cause of primary hyperaldosteronism is an **aldosterone-producing adenoma**, accounting for about 70% to 80% of all cases.

Another 20% to 30% of cases are caused by **idiopathic** hyperaldosteronism resulting from either bilateral (common) or unilateral (rare) hyperplasia of the zona glomerulosa of the adrenal cortex.

Other rare disorders include adrenocortical carcinoma, which may overproduce aldosterone, and the syndrome of glucocorticoid-remediable aldosteronism (GRA), sometimes called *dexamethasone-suppressible hyperaldosteronism.*

3. Is edema a sign of primary hyperaldosteronism?

No. Edema is seen typically in some states of secondary hyperaldosteronism (see later). When a patient with primary hyperaldosteronism has edema, it is prudent to search for another cause of the edema.

4. Why don't patients with primary hyperaldosteronism get edema?

The lack of edema results from an escape phenomenon, a spontaneous diuresis that returns sodium excretion to the level of intake and partially lowers the extracellular fluid volume toward normal. **Aldosterone escape** is thought to be mediated by an initial volume expansion that leads to increased atrial stretch and secretion of atrial natriuretic peptide with subsequent natriuresis.

5. Is the serum sodium concentration altered in primary hyperaldosteronism?

Although aldosterone causes sodium retention, the serum sodium concentration typically ranges within the upper limits of normal (i.e., 143–147 mEq/L). The osmostat that normally regulates antidiuretic hormone secretion is sensitive to small changes in osmolarity, which is not influenced by distal tubular sodium absorption. The mild persistent volume expansion typical of patients with primary hyperaldosteronism may reset the osmostat, altering antidiuretic hormone secretion so that mild hypernatremia can occur.

6. How does hypokalemia interfere with the diagnosis of primary hyperaldosteronism?

Potassium is one of the factors that regulates aldosterone excretion by exerting a direct effect on the zona glomerulosa. Hypokalemia inhibits the secretion of aldosterone. Conversely, **potassium loading** may stimulate aldosterone secretion. When evaluating a patient for suspected primary hyperaldosteronism, it is important to assess aldosterone secretion after hypokalemia has been corrected and potassium supplements have been discontinued.

7. Describe the best tests to establish the diagnosis of primary hyperaldosteronism.

When inappropriate kaliuresis (24-hour urinary potassium > 30 mEq in the presence of hypokalemia) has been confirmed, measurement of **24-hour urine aldosterone** after sodium loading has a high sensitivity and specificity. Sodium loading can be achieved by infusion of 2 L of normal saline over 4 hours or by oral sodium intake > 250 mEq daily for 3 days. Urine aldosterone levels normally fall to < 14 μg/d (39 nmol/L/d) in response to sodium loading. Similarly the serum aldosterone concentration falls to < 5 to 6 ng/dL after sodium loading. Values > 10 ng/dL indicate hyperaldosteronism.

Concomitant assessment of **plasma renin activity** (PRA) is necessary to distinguish primary from secondary hyperaldosteronism. PRA is suppressed in primary hyperaldosteronism and generally is elevated in secondary cases. Single random serum samples for aldosterone or urinary measurements without sodium loading are variable and unreliable.

Assessment of the **plasma aldosterone-to-renin ratio** can be done without special dietary preparation and has a high sensitivity and specificity. It is a good screening test for primary hyperaldosteronism. The mean value for the ratio in normal subjects or in patients with essential hypertension is 4 to 5, whereas the ratio is > 30 in most patients with primary hyperaldosteronism. Although PRA may be low in some patients with essential hypertension (**low-renin essential hypertension**), the plasma aldosterone-to-renin ratio remains normal. All tests of the renin-angiotensin-aldosterone system need to be performed after correction of hypokalemia and after cessation of diuretics, angiotensin-converting enzyme inhibitors, or β-blockers for > 2 weeks and cessation of spironolactone for > 4 weeks.

8. Why is it important to distinguish aldosterone-producing adenomas (or rarely carcinoma) from adrenal hyperplasia?

Their treatments differ. **Adenomas** should be removed surgically. **Hyperplasia**, which generally presents with milder degrees of aldosterone hypersecretion and less hypokalemia, does not respond to surgery and should be treated medically.

9. Describe the best biochemical tests to establish the specific cause of primary hyperaldosteronism.

Normally, plasma aldosterone levels rise after a person assumes an upright posture. In patients with aldosterone-producing adenomas, aldosterone secretion is sensitive to **adrenocorticotropin hormone (ACTH)**. Because of diurnal variations in ACTH secretion, plasma aldosterone levels paradoxically decrease between 8 AM and noon, despite upright posture. Plasma levels of 18-hydroxycorticosterone are elevated (> 100 ng/dL) after an overnight bed rest. In hyperaldosteronism resulting from adrenal hyperplasia, aldosterone secretion is sensitive to angiotensin, and the expected rise of aldosterone levels after assumption of an upright posture occurs. Plasma 18-hydroxycorticosterone levels after an overnight bed rest are lower (< 50 ng/dL).

10. List the radiologic tests that are helpful in the diagnosis of primary hyperaldosteronism.

CT

MRI

Radionuclide scintigraphy

11. Discuss the accuracy and problems associated with the radiologic tests for primary hyperaldosteronism diagnosis.

Patients with an adrenal adenoma or carcinoma have a unilateral adrenal mass. **CT** and **MRI** have sensitivities and specificities of 50% to 100%. The major problem is that some aldosterone-producing tumors are quite small (< 1 cm) and may be missed. In some patients, nodular hyperplasia may masquerade as a unilateral mass. Some patients have adrenal *incidentalomas*, most of which are benign, hormonally inactive adrenal cortical adenomas. **Radionuclide scintigraphy** using radiolabeled cholesterol derivatives has the advantage of being a functional test so that incidentalomas can be excluded with few false-positive results. The limited availability of the appropriate radionuclides has prevented widespread use of this technology. The accuracy of radionuclide scintigraphy is similar to that of CT and MRI.

12. What is the definitive diagnostic test for aldosterone-producing adenoma?

Bilateral adrenal venous sampling. Definitive diagnosis is made when one adrenal vein has 10 times the aldosterone concentration of the contralateral vein. There is little difference between the two sides in patients with adrenal hyperplasia. Catheterization of the adrenal veins, particularly on the right side, can be technically difficult, however, so that the test is not always feasible.

13. How effective is surgical treatment for aldosterone-producing adenomas?

Surgery is successful in removing aldosterone-producing adenomas and generally results in reduction of aldosterone secretion and correction of hypokalemia. Surprisingly, although the blood pressure almost always decreases to some degree, mild-to-moderate hypertension persists in 40% of patients. This persistent hypertension likely reflects underlying essential hypertension in some patients and the irreversible consequences of prolonged preoperative hypertension in most. The development of laparoscopic approaches to adrenal surgery has been a major technical advance in the field, but the best results are seen in experienced hands.

14. How effective is medical therapy?

Idiopathic adrenal hyperplasia may be a variant of essential hypertension mediated by higher than normal sensitivity of the zona glomerulosa to angiotensin II. Consequently, for patients with adrenal hyperplasia, medical management is preferred, using potassium-sparing diuretics (e.g., spironolactone or amiloride) with the addition of angiotensin-converting enzyme inhibitors if necessary. Some calcium channel blockers (e.g., nifedipine) inhibit aldosterone and may be effective adjunctively. For patients with aldosterone-producing adenomas who are not good surgical candidates or who decline surgery, treatment with spironolactone is effective in treating the hypertension and the hypokalemia.

15. Discuss GRA.

Glucocorticoid-remediable aldosteronism (GRA) is a rare disorder, with auto-somal-dominant inheritance, that results from a mutation that causes the formation of a chimeric (hybrid) gene. This gene contains the fusion of nucleotide sequences of the 11β-hydroxylase and aldosterone synthase genes so that the regulatory elements of the former control the latter. Because the 11β–hydroxylase gene is regulated by ACTH, aldosterone secretion in patients with GRA is stimulated by ACTH. Presence of the chimeric gene in the zona fasciculata (where cortisol usually is produced) leads to excessive production of aldosterone and secondary suppression of renin production that decreases the production of aldosterone in the zona glomerulosa. GRA is associated with hemorrhagic strokes at an early age, primarily as a result of ruptured intracranial aneurysms. This may reflect the influence of congenital hypertension during the early stages of cerebrovascular development.

16. How is GRA diagnosed?

When GRA is suspected on the basis of a family history of hypertension and hypokalemia, suppression of aldosterone levels by dexamethasone (0.25–0.5 mg/d) and the absence of a tumor on imaging studies helps to confirm the diagnosis.

17. What is the treatment for GRA?

Corticosteroids, which provide negative feedback on ACTH secretion, suppress the function of the chimeric gene.

18. What are some causes of mineralocorticoid excess–like states besides primary hyperaldosteronism?

When patients exhibit the manifestations of mineralocorticoid excess in the presence of low serum or urinary aldosterone levels, there is likely to be a nonaldosterone mineralocorticoid at work. This can occur in patients taking **fludrocortisone** (Florinef). Increased levels of deoxycorticosterone can occur in rare patients with deoxycorticosterone-producing adenomas and with some types of **congenital adrenal hyperplasia** (see Chapter 12). In some circumstances, the glucocorticoid **cortisol** acts as a mineralocorticoid. Cortisol binds as avidly as aldosterone to the mineralocorticoid receptor, but normally this cortisol is converted to cortisone in those tissues by the enzyme, 11β–hydroxysteroid dehydrogenase. Cortisone has little affinity for the mineralocorticoid receptor. This deactivation mechanism may be deficient in patients with deficiency of the dehydrogenase enzyme (the syndrome of **apparent mineralocorticoid excess**) or in patients who ingest **licorice**. The active factor in licorice is glycyrrhetinic acid, a steroid that inhibits the 11b–hydroxysteroid dehydrogenase enzyme. The deactivation mechanism may be overwhelmed by the extremely high cortisol levels sometimes found in the **ectopic ACTH syndrome**. **Liddle's syndrome** is a rare autosomal dominant condition involving a mutation in the gene for the collecting tubule sodium channel. This results in sodium reabsorption in the collecting tubules and, in most cases, augmented potassium secretion, resulting in a syndrome sometimes referred to as **pseudohyperaldosteronism** (see Chapter 13).

19. Did you say licorice?

Yes, but only genuine **black** licorice, not the fake black stuff or the red stuff.

20. Define secondary hyperaldosteronism.

Secondary hyperaldosteronism occurs whenever renin production is increased primarily. Conditions resulting in secondary hyperaldosteronism include disorders associated with extracellular volume depletion, malignant hypertension, and the common edema-forming states (congestive heart failure, cirrhosis, nephrotic syndrome). These conditions may or may not be associated with hypertension. Treatment is directed toward correcting the underlying condition.

BIBLIOGRAPHY

1. Barvo EL: Primary aldosteronism: Issues in diagnosis and management. Endocrinol Metab Clin North Am 23:2171–2283, 1994.
2. Botero-Velez M, Curtis JJ, Warnock DO: Liddle's syndrome revisited: A disorder of sodium reabsorption in the distal tubule. N Engl J Med 330:178, 1994.
3. Dluhy RG, Lifton RP: Glucocorticoid-remediable aldosteronism. Endocrinol Metab Clin North Am 23:285–297, 1994.

11. PHEOCHROMOCYTOMA

Uday A. Desai, M.D.

1. What is pheochromocytoma?

The term *pheochromocytoma* is derived from the Greek, *phios* ("dusky") and *chroma* ("color"). Pheochromocytoma is a catecholamine-producing tumor arising from the chromaffin cells of the sympathetic nervous system that are distinguished by their embryonic derivation from the primitive neural crest cells and their uptake of chromium salts. Most pheochromocytomas arise from the **adrenal gland**. About 10% arise from extra-adrenal sites, such as the carotid body and abdominal sympathetic ganglia, including the organ of Zuckerkandl, which consists of ganglia at the bifurcation of the aorta.

2. What is the incidence of pheochromocytoma?

It is responsible for < 0.1% of all patients with hypertension.

3. What catecholamines are produced by pheochromocytoma?

Norepinephrine is the catecholamine secreted predominantly by most pheochromocytomas. Tumors that predominantly secrete epinephrine are less common and more often are malignant or extra-adrenal in location. Synthesis of catecholamines begins with the amino acid **tyrosine** derived either from the diet or from hydroxylation of phenylalanine (see figure).

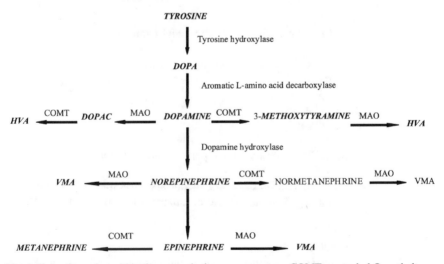

Metabolism of tyrosine within the sympathetic nervous system. COMT = catechol O-methyltransferase; MAO = monoamine oxidase; HVA = homovanillic acid; VMA = vanillylmandelic acid; DOPA = dihydroxyphenylalanine; DOPAC = dihydroxyphenylacetic acid.

Pheochromocytomas store and secrete a variety of **peptides:** endogenous opioids, endothelin, erythropoietin, parathyroid hormone–related protein, neuropeptide Y and chromogranin-A. Little is known about the mechanism of hormone release from pheochromocytomas, but changes in blood flow and necrosis within the tumor may be the cause in some cases.

4. Describe the clinical manifestations of pheochromocytoma.

The most common finding is **hypertension**, which occurs in > 90% of patients and which is paroxysmal in character in 20% to 25% of cases. Paroxysmal episodes of hypertension typically are associated with other signs and symptoms of catecholamine excess, such as tremor, tachycardia, hyperhydrosis, headache, and pupillary dilation. **Orthostatic hypotension** may occur as a result of decreased sympathetic reflexes reflecting down-regulation of adrenergic receptors. **Weight loss** may result from chronic hypermetabolism.

5. List the five Hs associated with pheochromocytoma.
- **H**ypertension
- **H**eadache
- **H**ypermetabolism
- **H**yperhydrosis
- **H**yperglycemia

6. What is the rule of 10%?
Each of the following accounts for 10% of all pheochromocytomas:
- Bilateral (in adrenal gland)
- Extra-adrenal
- Malignant
- Familial (associated with multiple endocrine neoplasia [MEN] syndromes)
- Pediatric

7. List conditions that are associated with pheochromocytoma.
Familial
1. von Recklinghausen's disease (neurofibromatosis)
2. Tuberous sclerosis
3. Sturge-Webber syndrome
4. von Hippel–Lindau disease
5. Ataxia telangiectasia
6. MEN syndrome
   a. MEN type 2: Pheochromocytoma, parathyroid adenoma, medullary carcinoma of thyroid
   b. MEN type 3: Pheochromocytoma, medullary carcinoma of thyroid, mucosal neuromas, abdominal gangliomas, marfanoid body habitus

Nonfamilial
1. Cholelithiasis
2. Cushing's syndrome
3. Carney's triad (gastric leiomyosarcoma, pulmonary chondroma, and paragangliomas)
4. Renal artery stenosis

8. List some clinical clues to the diagnosis of pheochromocytoma.
1. Sustained or paroxysmal hypertension associated with the triad of headache, palpitations, and diaphoresis

2. Hypertension and family history of pheochromocytoma
3. Refractory hypertension, especially if associated with weight loss
4. Sinus tachycardia
5. Orthostatic hypotension
6. Recurrent arrhythmias
7. Features of MEN type 2 or 3
8. Hypertensive crises during surgery or anesthesia
9. Pressor response to β-blocker
10. Incidentally discovered adrenal mass

9. List the causes of death in patients with pheochromocytoma.
- Myocardial infarction
- Arrhythmias
- Cerebrovascular accident
- Renal failure
- Dissecting aortic aneurysm

10. Elaborate on the biochemical screening for pheochromocytoma.
Measurement of catecholamines and their metabolites in the plasma and urine is recommended for screening. Small tumors may exhibit rapid turnover rates and release mainly unmetabolized catecholamines. Larger tumors often exhibit slower turnover rates associated with higher concentrations of catecholamine metabolites in plasma and urine. Resting plasma catecholamine concentrations > 2000 pg/ml suggest a pheochromocytoma, whereas values < 500 pg/ml are normal. Intermediate values (500–2000 pg/ml) are equivocal and mandate additional testing if clinical suspicion is high. Urine screening consists of measuring metanephrines, vanillylmandelic acid, and free catecholamines in a 24-hour urine collection.

11. Summarize diagnosis and treatment of pheochromocytoma.

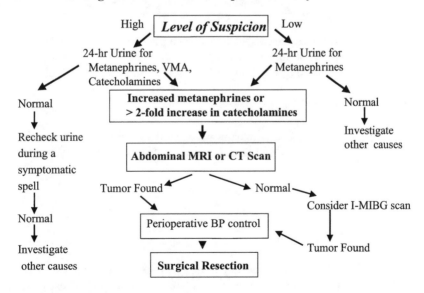

Diagnosis and treatment of pheochromocytoma.

12. What are the potential sources of error in chemical screening tests?

Plasma catecholamines levels may be elevated falsely with any kind of stress. In patients with paroxysmal hypertension, urinary concentration of catecholamines and their metabolites may be normal if the 24-hour urine is collected when the patient is normotensive and asymptomatic. Drugs also can alter levels.

13. Which drugs alter the measured levels of catecholamines and metabolites?

INCREASE	DECREASE
Tricyclic antidepressants	Metyrosine
Amphetamine	Methylglucamine
β-Blocker (labetalol, sotalol)	
Benzodiazepines	
L-Dopa, methyldopa	
Ethanol	
Withdrawal from clonidine	

14. What tests should be performed in equivocal cases?

TEST	RATIONALE
Regitine (phentolamine test)	Phentolamine is an α-blocker, and a reduction in blood pressure suggests catecholamine excess; not very sensitive or specific
Glucagon stimulation test	Glucagon stimulates catecholamine release; associated with a risk of precipitating a hypertensive crisis
Clonidine suppression test	Clonidine decreases central sympathetic outflow but does not suppress autonomous production by a tumor; failure to suppress plasma norepinephrine by > 50% after administration of clonidine suggests a pheochromocytoma

15. What imaging studies are used to localize a pheochromocytoma?

CT and MRI of the abdomen are imaging studies of choice. I-metaiodobenzyl-guanidine (MIBG) scintigraphy employs an isotope with affinity for chromaffin tissue and can be used to detect extra-adrenal tumors or to confirm that an adrenal mass is a pheochromocytoma.

16. What test can be used when imaging studies are equivocal?

Selective venous sampling of the vena cava at various levels can help to locate the tumor.

17. What is the treatment of choice for pheochromocytoma?

Surgical removal of the tumor is curative in 90% of cases.

18. Is medical therapy useful?

Mainly for perioperative management. Long-term medical therapy in form of a and β blockade or inhibition of catecholamine synthesis with α-methyl-paratyrosine can be used in patients with inoperable, recurrent, multicentric or malignant pheochromocytoma.

19. Describe perioperative management.

The goal of preoperative medical therapy is to control blood pressure (for 1–4 weeks before surgery) and to block the consequences of increased circulatory catecholamines. α-Blockers are the agents of choice, and phenoxybenzamine, a long-acting noncompetitive α-blocker, is preferred. The newer competitive/postsynaptic α-blockers (prazosin, terazosin) have a shorter action, provide incomplete α blockade, and are used less commonly. When tachycardia or arrhythmias persist, β-adrenergic blockade is indicated, but only after achieving α blockade to avoid unopposed α-receptor stimulation.

20. What clinical parameters should monitored in the postoperative period?

Persistent hypertension reflects:
• Fluid overload
• Return of autonomic reflexes
• Inadvertent ligation of renal artery
• Presence of residual tumor

Persistent hypotension reflects:
• Blood loss
• Altered vascular compliance
• Residual effect of preoperative α blockade

Hypoglycemia reflects:
• Removal of inhibitory effect of catecholamines on pancreatic islet cells
• Increased sensitivity of the β cells to glucose level after tumor removal
• Cessation of enflurane anesthesia—reactive increase in insulin

21. Discuss treatment for malignant pheochromocytoma.

Malignant pheochromocytoma accounts for < 10% of all pheochromocytomas. These are slow growing and poorly responsive to radiotherapy or chemotherapy. Surgical debulking may be necessary to decrease catecholamine synthesis. Radioactive MIBG has been used with some success to ablate primary and metastatic sites. α–Methyl-tyrosine has been tried in inoperable cases.

22. What is the prognosis of pheochromocytoma?

• 5-year survival > 95% in nonmalignant pheochromocytoma; < 50% in malignant pheochromocytoma
• Recurrence rate after surgery < 10% in nonmalignant pheochromocytoma
• Complete resection cures hypertension in approximately 75% of patients

In the remaining 25%, hypertension persists but is usually mild and well controlled with standard antihypertensive agents.

CONTROVERSY

23. How is pheochromocytoma managed during pregnancy?

Pheochromocytoma is a rare cause of hypertension during pregnancy. Diagnosis usually is based on the results of MRI and urinary catecholamines, vanillylmandelic acid, and metanephrine levels. Stimulation tests and MIBG scan are not considered safe in pregnancy. The optimal therapy is not well defined. The timing of surgery is controversial. Some authors recommend surgery if the fetus is previable (< 24 weeks of gestation) and medical management if pregnancy is advanced.

BIBLIOGRAPHY

1. Bravo EL: Pheochromocytoma: New concepts and future trends: Kidney Int 40:544–556,1991.
2. Kebew E, Duh QY: Benign and malignant pheochromocytoma: Diagnosis, treatment and follow up. Surg Oncol Clin N Am 7:765–789, 1998.
3. Russel WJ, Metcalf IR, Tonkin AL, Frewin DB: The preoperative management of pheochromocytoma. Anesth Intensive Care 26:196–200, 1998.
4. Venkata C, Ram S, Fierro-Carrion GA: Pheochromocytoma. Semin Nephrol 15:126–137, 1995.
5. Young WF: Pheochromocytoma and primary aldosteronism: Diagnostic approaches. Endocrinol Metab Clin North Am 26:801–827, 1997.

12. CUSHING'S SYNDROME AND CONGENITAL ADRENAL HYPERPLASIA

Beth A. Vogt, M.D.

1. What is Cushing's syndrome?

A symptom complex that reflects excessive tissue exposure to cortisol, first described in 1932.

2. Describe the most common clinical features of Cushing's syndrome.

Cushing's syndrome is characterized by **progressive physical changes**, often best appreciated in serial photographs. Central (truncal) obesity, moon facies, and a *buffalo hump* are classic physical findings. Additional physical findings include purple striae, plethora, ecchymoses, hypertrichosis, and muscle atrophy. Other features of Cushing's syndrome include emotional and cognitive changes, menstrual irregularity, glucose intolerance, and hypertension. **Growth retardation** is a universal finding in children with Cushing's syndrome.

3. How common is hypertension in Cushing's syndrome?

Although 80% of patients with Cushing's syndrome are hypertensive, Cushing's syndrome is a relatively rare cause of hypertension in children and adults.

4. Explain the mechanism of hypertension in patients with Cushing's syndrome.

Hypertension in patients with hypercortisolism is multifactorial in origin:
Excessive cortisol exposure increases **peripheral resistance** by:
  • Enhancing the effects of catecholamines and angiotensin II
  • Suppressing synthesis of endogenous vasodilatory agents, including nitric oxide and prostaglandins
Cortisol directly stimulates **sodium reabsorption** in the distal nephron, while indirectly increasing sodium reabsorption in the proximal nephron by enhancing the activity of various transporters.

Synthesis of certain **mineralocorticoids** is increased in adrenocorticotropin hormone (ACTH)—dependent types of Cushing's syndrome.

5. List the most common causes of Cushing's syndrome.
ACTH-dependent
  Pituitary adenoma
  Ectopic ACTH production (from other tumors)
  Ectopic corticotropin-releasing hormone (CRH) secretion
ACTH-independent
  Exogenous glucocorticoid administration
  Adrenal adenoma
  Adrenal adenocarcinoma
  Primary pigmented nodular adrenal hyperplasia

McCune-Albright syndrome
Macronodular adrenal disease
Hyperfunction of adrenal rest tissue

6. What is the difference between Cushing's syndrome and Cushing's disease?

Cushing's syndrome is a symptom complex that includes all patients with hypercortisolism.

Cushing's disease refers to a subset of Cushing's syndrome patients who have a pituitary adenoma as the cause of their hypercortisolism.

7. What are the best tests to confirm a diagnosis of Cushing's syndrome?

Plasma cortisol levels > 15 µg/dl in the afternoon or evening (in an unstressed patient) are suggestive of hypercortisolism.

Urinary free cortisol values > 100 µg/d are abnormal, and values > 400 µg/d (4 × normal) are suggestive of Cushing's syndrome.

Many clinicians use the **overnight dexamethasone suppression test** as a screen for Cushing's syndrome. Morning cortisol measurements < 5 µg/dl are appropriately suppressed and argue against a diagnosis of Cushing's syndrome.

8. What additional tests may be useful in identifying the cause of Cushing's syndrome?

Measurement of **plasma ACTH**. ACTH is suppressed in patients with ACTH-independent disease. ACTH is elevated in all cases of ACTH-dependent disease except in cases of ectopic ACTH production.

The dexamethasone suppression test, metyrapone stimulation test, and CRH stimulation test may help distinguish the origin of excessive corticosteroid effect.

Head and abdominal MRI may identify a pituitary or adrenal tumor.

9. List treatments for Cushing's syndrome.
- Adrenalectomy
- Pituitary adenoma resection
- Resection of tumor secreting ectopic ACTH

10. Is there a role for medical therapy?

Agents that **modulate ACTH release** (cyproheptadine, bromocriptine, valproic acid) or **inhibit cortisol production** (mitotane, trilostane, ketoconazole, aminoglutethimide, and metyrapone) may be useful while awaiting surgery or in treatment of patients who are not surgical candidates.

11. Should all obese patients with hypertension be evaluated for Cushing's syndrome?

No. Hypercortisolism should be considered in hypertensive patients who present with the body habitus and other characteristic clinical features.

12. Define congenital adrenal hyperplasia (CAH).

A family of autosomal recessive disorders in which there is a deficiency of one of the enzymatic activities necessary for cortisol synthesis (see figure).

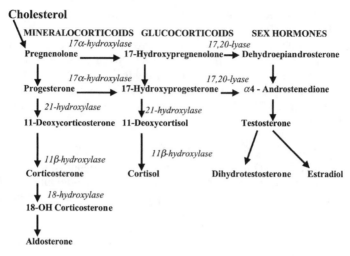

Pathways of steroid biosynthesis.

The reduction in cortisol synthesis leads to a loss of feedback inhibition of the hypothalamic-pituitary-adrenal axis, with excessive production of ACTH. Exposure to excessive ACTH leads to adrenal hyperplasia, overproduction of the adrenal steroids that do not require the deficient enzyme activity, and deficiency of steroids distal to the disrupted enzymatic step.

13. List the possible clinical manifestations of CAH.
- Abnormal fetal genital development
- Disturbance in sodium and potassium homeostasis (salt wasting or volume overload)
- Abnormal blood pressure regulation
- Postnatal consequences of sex steroid imbalance, including abnormal patterns of growth and maturation as well as impaired fertility

The specific clinical features depend on the specific enzyme deficiency.

14. What is the most common cause of CAH?
Deficiency of 21-hydroxylase activity, accounting for > 90% of cases.

15. What are other causes of CAH?
Deficiency of 11β-hydroxylase activity (5–8% of cases) is the second most common cause of CAH. Rare causes include 3β–hydroxysteroid dehydrogen deficiency, 17-hydroxylase deficiency, and lipoid CAH.

16. Which forms of CAH are associated with hypertension?
11β-hydroxylase deficiency and 17α-hydroxylase deficiency.

17. What about 21-hydroxylase deficiency?
The most common cause of CAH is not associated with hypertension. Patients with classic 21-hydroxylase deficiency have severe salt wasting with dehydration, hyponatremia, and hyperkalemia related to aldosterone deficiency.

18. Describe the pathophysiology of 11β-hydroxylase deficiency.

11β-hydroxylase (P450c11) is the mitochondrial enzyme responsible for the biosynthetic step immediately before cortisol production. More than 30 mutations have been identified on *CYP11B1*, the gene on chromosome 8, which encodes 11β-hydroxylase synthesis. Inadequate 11β-hydroxylation leads to inadequate cortisol production, excessive ACTH effect, and increased levels of the precursor deoxycorticosterone (DOC). Steroid synthesis is diverted to excessive androgen production.

19. What are the clinical features of 11β-hydroxylase deficiency?

1. 11β-Hydroxylase deficiency occurs in 1 in 100,000 individuals.

2. All affected females are born with some degree of masculinization of the external genitalia, including clitoromegaly and partial or complete fusion of the labioscrotal folds. Internal genitalia are normal.

3. Other symptoms of androgen excess that occur postnatally include rapid somatic growth with accelerated skeletal maturation, leading to premature closure of the epiphyses and short adult stature.

4. Mineralocorticoid excess leads to hypokalemic metabolic alkalosis in many patients.

5. Mild-to-moderate low-renin hypertension occurs in two thirds of patients, often beginning within the first few years of life.

20. Explain the mechanism of hypertension in patients with 11β-hydroxylase deficiency.

Hypertension is the result of volume expansion mediated by increased levels of DOC, a potent mineralocorticoid. Although DOC is a relatively weak mineralocorticoid, high levels produce significant sodium and water retention. Serum levels of DOC do not correlate entirely with the degree of hypertension, however, suggesting that other factors may be involved.

21. Describe the pathophysiology of 17α-hydroxylase deficiency.

17α-Hydroxylase (P450c17) is the enzyme responsible for the biosynthetic steps converting mineralocorticoids to glucocorticoids (17α-hydroxylase activity) and glucocorticoids to sex steroids (17,20-lyase activity). More than 20 mutations have been identified on *CYP17*, the gene on chromosome 10 that encodes 17α-hydroxylase synthesis. Abnormal enzyme activity can be manifested as isolated 17α-hydroxylase deficiency, 17,20-lyase deficiency, or combined 17α-hydroxylase/17,20-lyase deficiency. Inadequate 17α-hydroxylase activity leads to inadequate cortisol production, excessive ACTH effect, and increased levels of DOC. In contrast to in 11β-hydroxylase deficiency, sex steroid production is decreased.

22. What are the clinical features of 17α-hydroxylase deficiency?

1. Because patients with 17α-hydroxylase deficiency do not have excessive androgen synthesis, they tend to present later than patients do with 11β-hydroxylase deficiency.

2. Males may present with incomplete virilization and females may present with primary amenorrhea and sexual infantilism at the time of puberty.

3. Occasionally, genetic males with a female phenotype may present for evaluation of a hernia or inguinal mass.

4. Mineralocorticoid excess leads to hypokalemic metabolic alkalosis and mild-to-moderate low-renin hypertension.

23. Explain the mechanism of hypertension in patients with 17α-hydroxylase deficiency.

As in patients with 11β-hydroxylase deficiency, hypertension is the result of volume expansion mediated by increased levels of DOC. Serum levels of DOC do not correlate entirely with the degree of hypertension, suggesting that other factors may be involved.

24. How is CAH diagnosed?

Patients with various forms of CAH are diagnosed by their clinical features as well as plasma and urine steroid profiles. In general, the **ACTH stimulation test** results in marked elevation of precursor steroids proximal to the deficient enzyme. **Neonatal screening for 21-hydroxylase deficiency** is available in nearly 20 states in the United States as well as many countries worldwide. There is currently no screening program for the hypertensive forms of CAH because of the relative infrequency of these disorders. **Chorionic villus sampling** and **amniocentesis** may be useful in prenatal diagnosis of all forms of CAH in high-risk families.

25. In which hypertensive patients should CAH be considered in the differential diagnosis?

All hypertensive patients with:
- Hypokalemic metabolic alkalosis
- Abnormal external genitalia (virilized female, incompletely virilized male, or infantile female)
- History of infertility

26. Discuss the treatment for CAH.

In general, CAH is treated with long-term administration of **hydrocortisone** at a dose of 10 to 15 mg/m^2/d. This treatment provides negative feedback to the pituitary, which decreases ACTH synthesis and corrects excessive mineralocorticoid and sex steroid synthesis. In salt-wasting forms of CAH, such as 21-hydroxylase deficiency, administration of **fludrocortisone** (Florinef) and **sodium chloride** is necessary. Virilized females with 11β-hydroxylase deficiency require **surgical correction** of the external genitalia. **Sex steroids** are necessary in patients with hypogonadotropic hypogonadism, such as in 17α-hydroxylase deficiency. Maternal treatment with **dexamethasone** during pregnancy has been successful in preventing abnormal fetal genital development. New treatments may include **gene therapy**, although to date this approach has been confined to adrenocortical cell lines and animal models.

27. What are the antihypertensive agents of choice in the treatment of hypertension in patients with CAH?

- Potassium-sparing diuretics (spironolactone or amiloride)
- Calcium channel blockers

28. Which antihypertensive agents should be avoided?

Because renin is suppressed, angiotensin-converting enzyme inhibitors are unlikely to be effective. Thiazide diuretics should be avoided because of the possibility of aggravating hypokalemia.

BIBLIOGRAPHY

1. Brem A: Insights into glucocorticoid-associated hypertension. Am J Kidney Dis 37:1–10, 2001.
2. Carlson A, Obeid J, Kanellopoulou N, et al: Congenital adrenal hyperplasia: Update on prenatal diagnosis and treatment. J Steroid Biochem Mol Biol 69:19–29, 1999.
3. Levine L: Congenital adrenal hyperplasia. Pediatr Rev 21:159–170, 2000.
4. Pang S: Congenital adrenal hyperplasia. Endocrinol Metab Clin North Am 26:853–891, 1997.
5. Stratakis C, Rennert O: Congenital adrenal hyperplasia: Molecular genetics and alternative approaches to treatment. Crit Rev Clin Lab Sci 36:329–363, 1999.
6. White P: Inherited forms of mineralocorticoid hypertension. Hypertension 28:927–936, 1996.

13. OTHER FORMS OF SECONDARY HYPERTENSION

Donald E. Hricik, M.D.

1. Name some unusual causes of secondary hypertension.

Coarctation of the aorta	Obstructive sleep apnea
Thyroid disorders	Drug-induced hypertension
Hyperparathyroidism	Liddle's syndrome

2. What is coarctation of the aorta?

A congenital narrowing of the aorta, usually occurring somewhere between the aortic arch and the abdominal aorta. Although coarctation of the aorta is the fourth leading cause of congenital heart disease, it is a relatively uncommon cause of hypertension in childhood (see Chapter 14). The diagnosis always should be considered, however, because repair of the coarctation can correct hypertension and exert a favorable affect on patient survival.

3. How is coarctation of the aorta diagnosed?

Findings on physical examination include **diminished femoral pulses** and a **systolic pressure gradient** between BPs (BPs) obtained in the arms and legs. Despite this pressure gradient, many patients have hypertension below as well as above the aortic narrowing. A **loud systolic murmur** often can be heard in the posterior left interscapular area. When patients have developed collateral blood flow, continuous murmurs may be heard throughout the precordium.

Echocardiography with Doppler determinations can be used as a noninvasive test to localize the site of the coarcted segment. Definite diagnosis requires aortography.

4. What is a *3 sign?*

On the frontal projection of a chest radiograph, a thoracic coarctation may present as a **3 sign** consisting of the dilated proximal aorta, the coarctation itself, and poststenotic dilation.

Barium swallow may show indentations from the same structures, yielding a **reverse 3 sign**.

5. Explain the pathogenesis of hypertension in coarctation of the aorta.

1. Hypertension proximal to the coarcted segment may result from the high resistance to left ventricular flow.

2. Baroreceptors in the aortic arch may be *reset* to ensure that BP distal to the coarcted segment is adequate to perfuse distal organs.

3. Relatively low flow distal to the narrowing may result in renal hypoperfusion and lead to stimulation of the renin-angiotensin-aldosterone system.

Some patients develop persistent hypertension that is not corrected entirely by an otherwise adequate repair of the coarctation. Such patients exhibit evidence of abnormal baroreceptor activity and vascular reactivity in the upper extremities and respond well to conventional antihypertensive agents.

6. List treatments for coarctation of the aorta.
1. Surgery
   - Resection with end-to-end anastomosis
   - Flap angioplasty
   - Interposition of a synthetic tube graft
2. Balloon angioplasty

7. Discuss the prognosis of patients with coarctation of the aorta.
Untreated patients have a poor prognosis; 20% die within the first 2 decades of life, and 80% die before the age of 50. The 30-year survival is > 93% among patients in whom the coarctation is repaired before the age of 5. Patient survival is decreased among patients repaired at older ages. After successful repair, life expectancy often is reduced because patients may suffer from persistent hypertension, ischemic heart disease, and cerebrovascular disease.

8. Which thyroid disorders are associated with hypertension?
1. **Hyperthyroidism** (thyrotoxicosis) often is associated with an increased cardiac output and systolic hypertension. β–Blockers are effective in this setting, but definitive management consists of treating the underlying cause of excessive thyroid hormone production.

2. **Hypothyroid** patients exhibit a threefold increase in the incidence of hypertension. The pathophysiology is poorly understood. BP is lowered in most patients after adequate thyroid hormone replacement.

3. **Medullary carcinoma** of the thyroid does not cause hypertension but may be associated with pheochromocytoma (see Chapter 11) in patients with multiple endocrine neoplasia syndrome types IA and IIB.

9. What mechanism accounts for hypertension in patients with primary hyperparathyroidism?
Hypertension most often is attributed to the vasoconstrictive effects of the associated **hypercalcemia**. Hypertension is not observed routinely, however, in patients with other disorders associated with hypercalcemia (e.g., sarcoidosis, multiple myeloma, carcinomatosis).

10. Why is the relationship between hyperparathyroidism and hypertension unclear?
Only 10% to 60% of patients with primary hyperparathyroidism exhibit hypertension, and remission of hypertension is variable after otherwise successful parathyroidectomy.

11. What is the link between sleep apnea and hypertension?
1. Obstructive sleep apnea occurs more commonly in hypertensive than in nonhypertensive individuals.

2. Apneic spells can be associated with transient and marked increases in BP that eventually may become sustained during waking hours.

3. Obstructive sleep apnea is associated independently with cardiovascular abnormalities, including arrhythmias, cor pulmonale, left ventricular hypertrophy, and myocardial infarction.

12. How should hypertension be managed in patients with sleep apnea?

Effective therapy of obstructive sleep apnea (e.g., **continuous positive airway pressure** or **uvuloplasty**) tends to reduce BP during sleep. The effects of therapy on daytime BP are variable, and conventional **antihypertensive medications** should be prescribed if daytime hypertension persists.

13. Name the mechanisms of action involved in hypertension caused by drugs or chemical substances.

Salt and water retention (e.g., corticosteroids, sex hormones, mineralocorticoids, nonsteroidal anti-inflammatory drugs [NSAIDs])

Sympathomimetic effects (e.g., decongestants, antidepressants, cocaine)

14. List some uncommon causes of drug-induced hypertension.
- **Glucagon** when administered to patients with pheochromocytoma
- **Naloxone** when administered as an opiate antagonist
- **Anesthetics** such as ketamine and desflurane
- Concomitant use of **sympathomimetic agents with β-blockers**—can lead to severe elevations of BP because of unopposed α-adrenergic vasoconstriction

15. What is general treatment for drug-induced hypertension?

Drug-induced hypertension is managed optimally by discontinuation of the offending agent. If this is not possible, pharmacologic therapy may be needed.

16. List some specific initial treatment strategies.

DRUG/SUBSTANCE	INITIAL TREATMENT
Steroids (corticosteroids, mineralocorticoids, sex hormones)	Diuretics
NSAIDs	Diuretics
Antidepressants (monoamine oxidase inhibitors, tricyclics, serotonin antagonists)	α-Blockers
Nasal decongestants	α-, β-Blockers
Cocaine	α-Blockers
Cyclosporine	Calcium antagonists/diuretics

17. Define Liddle's syndrome.

Liddle's syndrome (also known as **pseudohyperaldosteronism**) is a rare disorder that results from genetic mutations that constitutively increase the passive reabsorption of sodium through apical channels in distal tubular cells. Patients present with volume-mediated hypertension, hypokalemia, and metabolic alkalosis. In contrast to patients with primary hyperaldosteronism (see Chapter 10), however, renin and aldosterone levels are suppressed because of the accompanying volume expansion.

18. How is Liddle's syndrome treated?

With drugs that inhibit sodium absorption in the distal nephron (e.g., amiloride or triamterene).

19. What about spironolactone?

Because the syndrome does not involve mineralocorticoid excess, spironolactone is of no benefit.

CONTROVERSY

20. Discuss alcohol and hypertension.

Epidemiologic studies indicate a consistent association between alcohol consumption and hypertension. Alcohol may stimulate the sympathetic nervous system or inhibit natural vasodilators. If the patient consumes > 2 drinks a day (a standard drink contains about 14 g of ethanol), the higher the alcohol intake, the higher the BP. The effects of alcohol are independent of age, ethnicity, or body weight. A reduction in alcohol consumption usually is associated with a decrease in BP. Low levels of alcohol intake (< 2 drinks a day) are associated with a reduced risk of atherothrombotic events, such as myocardial infarction and stroke.

BIBLIOGRAPHY

1. Clyburn BE, DiPette DJ: Hypertension induced by drugs and other substances. Semin Nephrol 15:72–86, 1995.
2. Levinson PD, Millman RP: Causes and consequences of blood pressure alterations in obstructive sleep apnea. Arch Intern Med 151:455–462, 1991.
3. Noda A, Okada T, Hayashi H, et al: 24-hour ambulatory blood pressure variability in obstructive sleep apnea syndrome. Chest 103:1343–1347, 1993.
4. Saito I, Saruta T: Hypertension in thyroid disorders. Endocrinol Metab Clin North Am 23:379–386, 1994.
5. Stewart AB, Ahmed R, Travill CM, Newman CG: Coarctation of the aorta: Life and health 20–44 years after surgical repair. Br Heart J 69:65–70, 1993.

14. CHILDHOOD HYPERTENSION

Ira D. Davis, M.D.

1. How is hypertension defined in children?

Hypertension is based on the normal distribution of systolic and diastolic blood pressure (BP) in the general population for children of comparable age, weight, and height.

2. How is BP in children classified?

High normal BP: BP between 90th and 95th percentile
Significant hypertension: BP between 95th and 99th percentile
Severe hypertension: BP > 99th percentile

3. When should BP be checked in children?

The American Academy of Pediatrics recommends that annual BP screening begin at 3 years of age.

4. Is there a proper cuff size necessary for measuring BP in children?

The size of the inner bladder width is crucial because overestimation of BP occurs when the cuff is too small, whereas underestimation of BP occurs when the cuff is too large. The bladder length should encompass the circumference of the upper arm completely and should cover at least 75% of the upper arm length between the antecubital fossa and the axilla. When measuring the BP, the arm should be supported with the antecubital fossa at the level of the heart.

5. Does essential hypertension occur in children?

Essential hypertension accounts for approximately 10% to 20% of cases of hypertension in children < 10 years old. It accounts for about 35% of cases of hypertension in adolescents.

6. What is the incidence of hypertension in newborns?

- 0.2% to 3% in all newborns
- > 1% in premature newborns and high-risk newborns

7. What is the primary cause of hypertension in newborn infants?

Renovascular disease associated with renal arterial thromboemboli or renal artery stenosis

8. List other causes of hypertension in newborns.

- Coarctation of the aorta
- Congenital renal malformations, such as obstructive uropathy or polycystic kidney disease
- Bronchopulmonary dysplasia

9. List the most common causes of hypertension in infants through preschool-age children.

Hypertension secondary to:
• Renal parenchymal disease
• Renal artery stenosis
• Coarctation of the aorta

10. What are the most common causes of hypertension in children 6 to 10 years old?

Hypertension secondary to renal parenchymal disease or renal artery stenosis.

11. What is the most common cause of secondary hypertension in adolescents?

Renal parenchymal disease, including acute or chronic forms of glomerulonephritis and renal scarring associated with a remote history of pyelonephritis.

12. List clinical characteristics that are associated commonly with essential hypertension.

• Mild BP elevations (often to > 95th percentile, with significant variability in measurements)
• Strong family history
• Obesity

13. What features of the medical history should be emphasized when evaluating a child with hypertension?

1. A careful family history including the age of onset of hypertension and the presence of complications, such as myocardial infarction, kidney failure, heart failure, stroke, and peripheral vascular disease, in first-degree and second-degree relatives is essential.

2. The patient's growth pattern and neonatal history should be assessed.

3. Patients should be questioned regarding the intake of foods and medications (including over-the-counter and illicit drugs) that cause elevations in BP, such as caffeine, nicotine, sodium, sympathomimetics, steroids, cocaine, and amphetamines.

4. Patients should be questioned about symptoms of severe hypertension (see later).

14. What are the symptoms of hypertension in children?

1. Children with **essential hypertension** or **mildly elevated BP owing to secondary causes** are usually asymptomatic.

2. **Severe hypertension** may be associated with headaches, epistaxis, dizziness, blurred vision, nausea, changes in mental status, or seizures.

3. **Neonates** with hypertension may present with poor feeding, irritability, lethargy, respiratory distress, seizures, or apnea.

15. List the important features of the physical examination when evaluating a child with hypertension.

1. Growth assessment
2. Four extremity BP measurements for evidence of coarctation of the aorta

3. Funduscopic examination and a careful neurologic examination
4. Neck examination for evidence of thyromegaly
5. Cardiopulmonary examination for evidence of congestive heart failure or murmurs
6. Abdominal examination for masses or bruits
7. Skin examination looking for manifestations of rheumatologic diseases (e.g., systemic lupus erythematosus) or neurocutaneous syndromes (e.g., neurofibromatosis or tuberous sclerosis)
8. Genitalia

16. Describe the initial approach to the laboratory evaluation of hypertension in children.

All patients with hypertension require a urinalysis, serum chemistries, blood urea nitrogen, and creatinine determination.

A **fasting lipid profile** should be checked in patients with suspected essential hypertension.

Patients with suspected secondary hypertension owing to urologic abnormalities or pyelonephritis should have a **urine culture**.

Children with severe hypertension and all children <13 years old should undergo a **renal ultrasound**.

Patients with tachycardia or thyromegaly should have thyroid function studies.

Echocardiography should be performed in patients with BP >95th percentile and when pharmacotherapy is being considered.

17. List nonpharmacologic approaches to the treatment of hypertension in children.
• Weight reduction
• Aerobic exercise
• Dietary modifications (low salt and low fat)

18. When are pharmacologic approaches necessary in treating childhood hypertension?
1. Presence of significant hypertension unresponsive to nonpharmacologic approaches
2. Presence of symptoms
3. Presence of end-organ injury evidenced by increased left ventricular mass or left ventricular dysfunction on echocardiogram
4. Presence of severe hypertension.

19. What is the goal of treatment?
To reduce BP < 95th percentile

BIBLIOGRAPHY

1. Bartosh SM, Aronson AJ: Childhood hypertension: An update on etiology, diagnosis, and treatment. Pediatr Clin North Am 46:235–252, 1999.
2. Coody DK, Yetman RJ, Portman RJ: Hypertension in children. J Pediatr Health Care 9:3–11, 1995.
3. Flynn JT: Neonatal hypertension: Diagnosis and management. Pediatr Nephrol 14:332–334, 2000.

4. National High Blood Pressure Education Program Working Group on Hypertension Control in Children and Adolescents: Update on the 1987 task force report on high blood pressure in children and adolescents: A working group report from the National High Blood Pressure Education Program. Pediatrics 98:649–658, 1996.
5. Task Force on Blood Pressure Control in Children: Report of the second task force on blood pressure control in children—1987. Pediatrics 79:1–25, 1987.

15. HYPERTENSION IN PREGNANCY

Donald E. Hricik, M.D.

1. How does pregnancy normally influence systemic blood pressure (BP)?

During normal pregnancy, **systolic BP** changes little. **Diastolic BP** decreases by an average of 10 mm Hg by the 20th week of gestation and rises back to baseline levels in the third trimester. The normal decrease in BP early in gestation may mask the presence of antecedent chronic hypertension. Third-trimester hypertension generally is defined as a diastolic BP of ≥ 85 mm Hg.

2. What is the clinical importance of hypertension associated with pregnancy?

Hypertensive disorders are the most common medical complications of pregnancy, occurring in 20% of all cases. They are an important cause of maternal and fetal morbidity and mortality.

3. Classify the hypertensive disorders associated with pregnancy.
1. Preeclampsia/eclampsia
2. Chronic hypertension
3. Chronic hypertension with superimposed preeclampsia
4. Late or transient hypertension

4. Define preeclampsia/eclampsia.

Preeclampsia is a hypertensive disorder associated with proteinuria, edema, and sometimes coagulation and liver function abnormalities in pregnant women. The disorder occurs in 5% to 10% of all pregnancies and occurs most often in nulliparas, usually after the 20th week of gestation.

Preeclampsia can progress rapidly to **eclampsia**, a state characterized by seizures and often preceded by severe hypertension, headache, and hyperreflexia. The convulsive, eclamptic phase can occur suddenly in seemingly stable women with mild BP elevations. Third-trimester hypertension should be regarded and treated as preeclampsia until proven otherwise.

5. Define chronic hypertension associated with pregnancy.

Most women in this category have essential hypertension, but secondary forms of hypertension always merit consideration. Patients with preexisting hypertension may exhibit elevated BP's during the first two trimesters. Women with pregestational hypertension are more prone to superimposed preeclampsia (category 3 in the aforementioned classification scheme).

6. Define late or transient hypertension associated with pregnancy.

The development of hypertension in the third trimester without associated proteinuria. Typically, maternal and fetal outcomes are normal, and BP returns to normal within 1 or 2 weeks of delivery.

7. Besides proteinuria, what are the other renal manifestations of preeclampsia?
Glomerular filtration rate decreases in preeclampsia in association with a renal lesion called **glomerular endotheliosis** and characterized by swelling of glomerular endothelial cells. Varying degrees of renal sodium retention contribute to the pathogenesis of edema in this disorder.

8. Describe the liver and coagulation abnormalities associated with preeclampsia.
Mild liver abnormalities are common. One variant of preeclampsia is characterized by severe liver dysfunction with markedly elevated **transaminase** levels. **Bilirubin** and **alkaline phosphatase** levels may be at least mildly elevated as well. Such patients often exhibit severe thrombocytopenia and evidence of microangiopathic hemolytic anemia. This form of preeclampsia (known as HELLP syndrome) is life-threatening and best managed by delivery or termination of the pregnancy.

9. How does eclampsia differ from hypertensive encephalopathy?
The **seizures** that occur in eclampsia have been attributed to intense cerebral vasoconstriction or to platelet thrombi that obstruct the cerebral microcirculation.
The **ophthalmologic** hallmarks of hypertensive encephalopathy (i.e., retinal hemorrhages, exudates, and papillary edema) are uncommon in eclampsia.

10. List conditions that can be confused with preeclampsia or eclampsia.
• Viral hepatitis
• Acute fatty liver of pregnancy
• Acute glomerulonephritis
• Thrombotic thrombocytopenic purpura/hemolytic-uremic syndrome
• Cerebral hemorrhage

11. List drugs that are preferred for the treatment of chronic hypertension associated with pregnancy.
• Methyldopa
• Hydralazine
• Labetalol

12. What drugs are not recommended or are contraindicated?
Atenolol and diuretics may be effective, but some studies suggest that these agents adversely affect fetal growth. **Angiotensin-converting enzyme inhibitors** are **contraindicated** in pregnancy because these drugs are associated with fetal growth retardation, congenital malformations, and neonatal renal failure.

CONTROVERSY

13. What is the pathophysiology of preeclampsia?
The vasculature of women with this disorder is intensely sensitive to endogenous pressor peptides and catecholamines as well as to exogenous infusions of pressors, such as angiotensin, norepinephrine, and vasopressin. This **vascular sensitivity** may be related to decreased levels of eicosanoids, such as prostaglandins

E and I. The hemodynamic profile of the preeclamptic woman is characterized by **volume depletion**, **salt retention**, and **edema**. One theory regarding pathogenesis is that a primary reduction in intravascular volume leads to placental hypoperfusion and release of pressor substances by the uterus. Other theories suggest that primary vasoconstriction leads secondarily to the observed reduction in plasma volume.

14. In a pregnant woman, how does one distinguish preeclampsia from underlying renal disease associated with hypertension?

Unless the woman's past medical history is well known, it can be difficult to distinguish these two entities. Many nephrologists are reluctant to perform a **kidney biopsy** in a pregnant woman to help make this differentiation. When doubt exists, it is probably prudent to manage the patient as though she has preeclampsia, particularly because underlying renal disease increases the risk of superimposed preeclampsia.

Because the clinical manifestations of preeclampsia resolve after delivery, persistence of proteinuria and hypertension several weeks after delivery strongly suggest underlying parenchymal renal disease.

15. Discuss management of preeclampsia.

Delivery is the ultimate cure but may not be feasible when preeclampsia occurs relatively early in pregnancy. There is disagreement about the need for bed rest, prolonged hospitalization, antihypertensive drug therapy, and anticonvulsant prophylaxis in women with **mild** preeclampsia; however, **bed rest** at home or in the hospital still is recommended commonly. Results of randomized trials designed to test the efficacy of antihypertensive drug therapy in preventing the progression of preeclampsia have yielded conflicting results.

In women with **severe** preeclampsia remote from term, the objective of treatment is to prevent cerebral complications. The aim of therapy is to keep the diastolic BP < 105 mm Hg (but not < 90 mm Hg). Intravenous **hydralazine** (administered as a 5-mg bolus every 20 minutes to a cumulative dose of 20 mg) is probably the drug of choice. Nifedipine and labetalol have been found to be safe and effective. Although routine **anticonvulsant prophylaxis** is controversial, intravenous magnesium sulfate is the treatment of choice for the treatment of eclamptic seizures and still is used by some obstetricians in a prophylactic manner in women with severe preeclampsia.

16. Are there other preventive modalities for preeclampsia?

Early single-center studies suggested that aspirin reduced the incidence and severity of preeclampsia. Subsequent large, randomized trials showed no benefit compared with placebo. **Aspirin** still may be useful in women with hypercoagulable states, such as the antiphospholipid antibody syndrome. Epidemiologic studies have suggested an inverse relationship between dietary calcium intake and the incidence of preeclampsia. The results of randomized trials comparing calcium supplementation with placebo suggest that **calcium supplements** may reduce the risk of gestational hypertension, but they have little impact on the incidence or severity of preeclampsia.

BIBLIOGRAPHY

1. Caroli G, Duley L, Belizan JM, Villar J: Calcium supplementation during pregnancy: A systemic review of randomized controlled trials. Br J Obstet Gynaecol 101:753–758, 1994.
2. Lindheimer MD: Preeclampsia–eclampsia 1996: Preventable? Have disputes on its treatment been resolved? Curr Opin Nephrol Hypertens 5:452–458, 1996.
3. Lindheimer MD, Katz AI: Hypertension in pregnancy. N Engl J Med 313:675–680, 1985.
4. Schobel HP, Fischer T, Heuszer K, et al: Preeclampsia—a state of sympathetic overactivity. N Engl J Med 335:1480–1485, 1996.
5. Sibai BM: Treatment of hypertension in pregnant women. N Engl J Med 335:257–265, 1996.

16. HYPERTENSION AFTER RENAL TRANSPLANTATION

Hany S. Y. Anton, M.D.

1. How common is hypertension after renal transplantation?

In the early 1980's the prevalence of hypertension in renal transplant recipients was 50–60%. However, since the introduction of cyclosporine, the prevalence has increased to 75–85%.

2. What are the causes of posttransplant hypertension?

Several mechanisms have been proposed to explain posttransplant hypertension:

- **Retained diseased native kidneys.** Increased renin production, increased sympathetic activity, and other mechanisms invoked as explanations for renal parenchymal hypertension (see Chapter 8) may play a role in transplant patients.
- **Recurrent or de novo disease in allograft.** Recurrent (e.g., focal glomerulosclerosis, IgA nephropathy, diabetic nephropathy) or de novo (e.g., membranous nephropathy, hemolytic uremic syndrome) renal diseases affecting the allograft can be associated with hypertension.
- **Acute and chronic rejection.** Hypertension is common in patients with acute renal allograft rejection and probably results from acute volume retention. Hypertension is also a common finding in patients with chronic allograft nephropathy (i.e., "chronic rejection"), although the mechanisms are not certain.
- **Donor factors.** With the increasing acceptance of organs from older or mildly hypertensive donors, it has been speculated that properties intrinsic to the donor kidney may be responsible for posttransplant hypertension.
- **Transplant renal artery stenosis.** The reported incidence of renal artery stenosis in transplanted kidneys ranges widely from 1 to 23%. This entity is of particular importance because of its reversibility. Clues to the presence of transplant renal artery stenosis include hypertension with worsening graft function, new onset or acute worsening of hypertension, and acute renal failure with the use of an angiotensin inhibitor. Unfortunately, none of these clinical scenarios is specific for renal artery stenosis. The gold standard for diagnosis is the conventional renal arteriogram or digital subtraction angiography. Because administration of toxic contrast agents is often a concern, noncontrast studies such as Doppler ultrasonography, CO_2 angiography, and magnetic resonance angiography are often performed initially. The sensitivities and specificities of the latter tests are highly operator-dependent.
- **Obesity and non-white ancestry** have been correlated with the prevalence and severity of posttransplant HTN.

3. What is the role of immunosuppressive drugs?

Hypertension is a common side effect of corticosteroid therapy and results, in part, from sodium retention and volume expansion. Withdrawal of steroid therapy results in improvement of blood pressure in most, and in cure of hypertension in approximately 15% of transplant recipients, but increases the risk of acute and chronic rejection. As mentioned in Question 1, the increased prevalence of posttransplant hypertension in the cyclosporine era suggests that this drug may play a role in the pathogenesis of posttransplant hypertension.

4. What are the putative mechanisms of cyclosporine-induced hypertension?
Several mechanisms have been invoked:
- Renal vasoconstriction
- Increased central sympathetic discharge
- Increased synthesis of endothelin
- Increased levels of thromboxane A_2

5. How does tacrolimus compare to cyclosporine in its effect on posttransplant hypertension?
The results of available studies are mixed. Part of the problem is that tacrolimus often is used with lower adjunctive doses of corticosteroids, so any perceived reduction in blood pressure may be the result of lower exposure to steroids and not to the beneficial effects of tacrolimus per se.

6. Should bilateral nephrectomy be performed in all candidates for kidney transplantation?
No. Several studies have shown a beneficial effect of bilateral nephrectomy on controlling posttransplant hypertension. However, some degree of hypertension may persist after removal of both kidneys. Furthermore, elimination of erythropoeitin production and of residual urine output from the native kidneys is a disadvantage to many patients with end-stage renal disease. With the availability of potent antihypertensive medications, bilateral nephrectomy is now performed rarely and is reserved for cases of severe, intractable hypertension. Nephrectomy is still performed occasionally in patients with large polycystic kidneys or in patients with vesicoureteral reflux and recurrent urinary tract infections. In such patients, control of posttransplant hypertension is an added benefit of the procedure.

7. What are the consequences of posttransplant hypertension?
In addition to the known increased risk of coronary artery disease and stroke, hypertension is a reliable predictor of poor graft survival in renal transplant recipients, especially in African Americans.

8. How should posttransplant hypertension be managed?
1. Lifestyle modification:
    - Cessation of smoking
    - Sodium restriction
    - Weight loss
    - Exercise
2. Medications:
    - **Calcium channel blockers** have been particularly effective in antagonizing the hypertensive and renal vasoconstrictive effect of cyclosporine, and are the drugs of choice in many transplant centers. Cautious use of diltiazem

and verapamil is recommended to avoid the elevations in cyclosporine, tacrolimus, or sirolimus levels, due to competition for cytochrome P450 enzymes involved in the metabolism of these drugs.

- **Diuretics** may be helpful in patients with sodium retention and fluid overload or hyperkalemia. Volume depletion is a potential complication of therapy. In addition, one should watch for hypomagnesemia, which may be exacerbated by the use of cyclosporine or tacrolimus.
- **Beta-blockers.** In addition to known beneficial effects in reducing mortality from coronary artery disease and congestive heart failure, beta blockers may be helpful in counteracting sympathetic overactivity due to cyclosporine.
- **Angiotensin inhibitors.** ACE inhibitors and angiotensin receptor blockers have traditionally been avoided as first-line agents for posttransplant agents for several reasons, including (1) the perception that this class of drugs is ineffective in controlling hypertension in transplant recipients, (2) concern about exacerbating hyperkalemia, and (3) concern about precipitating acute renal failure in patients with transplant renal artery stenosis. In addition, recent evidence suggests that these agents may interfere with erythropoiesis and cause anemia in kidney transplant recipients. Despite these concerns, there is growing interest in the use of angiotensin inhibitors to slow the progression of renal disease in patients at risk for chronic allograft nephropathy. Furthermore, recent head-to-head comparisons suggest that these agents can be just as effective as calcium channel blockers in controlling systemic posttransplant hypertension. Thus, increased use of angiotensin inhibitors for posttransplant hypertension can be anticipated in the next several years.
- **Centrally acting agents, alpha blockers, and vasodilators** are used adjunctively as second or third-line agents.

BIBLIOGRAPHY

1. Demme RA: Hypertension in the kidney transplant patient. Graft 4(4):248–255, 2001.
2. Hohage H, Bruckner D, Arlt M, et al: Influence of cyclosporine A and FK506 on 24h blood pressure monitoring in kidney transplant recipients. Clinical Nephrology 45:342–344, 1996.
3. Kasiske BL: Possible causes and consequences of hypertension in stable renal transplant patients. Transplantation 44(5):639–643, 1987.
4. Mange KC, Cizman B, Joffe M, Feldman HI: Arterial hypertension and renal allograft survival. JAMA 283:633–638, 2000.
5. Ponticelli C, Montagnino G, Aroldi C, et al: Hypertension after renal transplantation. Am J Kidney Dis 21(Suppl 2):73–78, 1993.
6. Schulak JA, Hricik DE: Steroid withdrawal after renal transplantation. Clin Transplant 8(2):211–216, 1994.
7. Stigant CE, Cohen J, Vivera M, Zaltzman JS: ACE inhibitors and angiotensin II antagonists in renal transplantation: An analysis of safety and efficacy. Am J Kidney Dis 35:58–63, 2000.

17. HYPERTENSION IN END-STAGE RENAL DISEASE

Mahboob Rahman, M.D., M.S.

1. What is the incidence of hypertension in patients with end-stage renal disease (ESRD)?

Of patients starting dialysis, 80% to 100% are hypertensive. In a random sample of patients undergoing long-term hemodialysis, 63% were hypertensive: 27%, stage 1; 25%, stage 2; 11%, stage 3 hypertension (as defined by the Sixth Joint National Committee).

2. Describe the problems associated with blood pressure (BP) measurement in hemodialysis patients.

BP can be measured before dialysis, after dialysis, or on days between dialysis treatments. The postdialysis BP is often lower than the predialysis readings, and BP gradually rises during the interdialytic period. The clinician faces the dilemma of determining which readings to target in efforts to control BP. Although controversial, most studies show that predialysis BP readings correlate best with hypertensive target organ damage.

3. What should be the goal of the treating physician in ESRD hypertension?

Optimizing predialysis BP.

4. Can ambulatory BP monitoring help in the management of hypertension in hemodialysis patients?

Given the variability of BP in hemodialysis patients, obtaining several readings over a 24- to 48-hour period may provide a better estimate of hypertension. The mean ambulatory BP correlates better with left ventricular hypertrophy than conventional BP measurement. The value of this technique in long-term management of hypertension has not been studied adequately.

5. Is hypertension an independent marker for mortality in hemodialysis patients?

In the general population, there is a strong association between high BP and mortality; however, in hemodialysis patients, such a relationship has **not** been shown. Low, not high, BP has been consistently predictive of mortality in these patients.

6. Explain the paradox of low BP being predictive of mortality in hemodialysis patients.

Patients with low BP may have other cardiac conditions (e.g., congestive heart failure) that increase their mortality. This confounds the relationship between BP and mortality in this population.

7. Is hypertension associated with specific morbidity in hemodialysis patients?
Yes, with worsening left ventricular hypertrophy, development of congestive heart failure, and increased hospitalizations.

8. List the pathophysiologic factors that contribute to hypertension in ESRD patients.
- Expansion of intravascular volume by sodium and fluid retention
- Activation of the renin-angiotensin system
- Increased sympathetic nervous system activity
- Imbalance in the endothelial production of vasodilator and vasoconstrictor substances

9. Discuss the relationship between erythropoietin therapy and BP.
The use of **recombinant human erythropoietin (rhEPO)** has improved significantly the management of anemia and quality of life in patients with ESRD. rhEPO therapy has been associated with **worsening of hypertension**. This may require additional antihypertensive drug therapy, but it is uncommon that rhEPO therapy has to be discontinued because of uncontrolled hypertension. The mechanisms underlying this pressor effect of rhEPO are not completely understood. Increased blood viscosity, reversal of hypoxic vasodilation as the hematocrit increases, and a direct effect of rhEPO on the vasculature have been postulated.

10. What should be the initial therapeutic intervention to control BP in hemodialysis patients?
Optimization of intravascular volume status. This can be achieved by limiting sodium intake and gradual removal of fluid on dialysis (**ultrafiltration**) until the patient reaches dry weight. Dry weight is defined clinically as the level below which further fluid removal would produce hypotension, muscle cramps, nausea, and vomiting. In many patients, BP can be controlled by achieving and maintaining patients close to their dry weight.

11. When should antihypertensive drug therapy be initiated?
When patients remain hypertensive despite attempts to achieve dry weight. In choosing among antihypertensive agents, consideration should be given to **co-existent conditions** (see Chapter 29).

12. List antihypertensive drugs that are effective in controlling BP in these patients.
- Calcium channel antagonists
- Angiotensin-converting enzyme inhibitors
- Centrally acting sympatholytic agents
- In some patients with **resistant hypertension**, treatment with **minoxidil** may be required.

13. How should you modify the doses of commonly used antihypertensive agents when used in ESRD patients?
Most dihydropyridine calcium channel antagonists (except nicardipine) do not require dosage modification in ESRD patients. The dosage of many other antihypertensive

agents need to be reduced for use in these patients. Standard sources, such as the *Physician's Desk Reference* or *Drug Prescribing in Renal Failure* from the American College of Physicians, should be consulted before prescribing antihypertensive drug therapy in patients with ESRD.

14. Is peritoneal dialysis associated with better control of BP than hemodialysis?

In peritoneal dialysis, fluid removal occurs more gradually and over longer periods of time. Some patients may be able to tolerate fluid removal better on peritoneal dialysis than hemodialysis, allowing them to reach their dry weight and achieve better BP control.

CONTROVERSY

15. Why does BP remain poorly controlled in many dialysis patients?

This may be due to inability to achieve **adequate fluid removal** and maintain patients at dry weight. Excessive interdialytic weight gains, poor compliance with dialysis regimen and medications, and inadequate prescription of antihypertensive drug therapy may contribute to inadequate BP control.

BIBLIOGRAPHY

1. Charra B, Bergstrom J, Scribner BH: Blood pressure control in dialysis patients: Importance of the lag phenomenon. Am J Kidney Dis 32:720–724, 1998.
2. Mailloux LU, Haley WE: Hypertension in the ESRD patient: Pathophysiology, therapy, outcomes, and future directions. Am J Kidney Dis 32:705–719, 1998.
3. Mailloux LU, Levey AS: Hypertension in patients with chronic renal disease. Am J Kidney Dis 32(5 suppl 3):S120–141, 1998.
4. Rahman M, Fu P, Sehgal AR, Smith MC: Interdialytic weight gain, compliance with dialysis regimen and age are independent predictors of blood pressure in hemodialysis patients. Am J Kidney Dis 35:257–265, 2000.

18. RESISTANT HYPERTENSION

Hany S. Y. Anton, M.D., and Michael C. Smith, M.D.

1. What is resistant hypertension?

Multiple definitions of resistant hypertension have been proposed over the last two decades. From a practical perspective, however, hypertension can be considered resistant when blood pressure remains greater than 140/90 mmHg despite an appropriate three-drug regimen, including a diuretic, prescribed at near-maximal doses. In patients with isolated systolic hypertension, resistance is defined as persistent systolic blood pressure greater than 160 mmHg with a similar regimen.

2. How common is resistant hypertension?

Fortunately, not common. Although resistant hypertension is more prevalent in referral populations, it occurs in only about 3% of the general hypertensive population.

3. List the causes of resistant hypertension.

Multiple classifications of resistant hypertension have been formulated. However, the most common causes are shown as follows.
- Patient Noncompliance
    Pharmacologic
    Dietary
- Physician Related
    Suboptimal medical regimen
    Pseudotolerance
    Drug interactions
    Pseudohypertension
- Office Hypertension
- Specific Pressor Mechanisms
    Secondary hypertension
    Reaction to antihypertensive therapy

4. How frequently is patient noncompliance a cause of resistant hypertension?

Several studies have estimated that lack of adherence to a properly prescribed medication regimen or failure to comply with dietary salt restriction accounts for 25–50% of resistant hypertension. Prescription of expensive medications, complicated drug regimens, and real or perceived adverse drug reactions contribute importantly to noncompliance with pharmacologic therapy. In addition, lack of instruction in, or lack of adherence to, a low-sodium diet (80–90 mmol/day) is often central to the development of resistant hypertension.

5. What physician-related issues contribute to the development of resistant hypertension?

Four are most important:

- Prescription of a suboptimal medical regimen
- Failure to appreciate the development of pseudotolerance
- Failure to identify drug interactions that blunt the effect of antihypertensive therapy
- Inability to recognize pseudohypertension

6. What constitutes a suboptimal medication regimen?

Inadequate antihypertensive regimens consist of those that prescribe drug combinations at suboptimal doses, use illogical drug combinations (e.g., two β-blockers), fail to include a diuretic, or employ thiazide diuretics in patients with creatinine clearances less than 30 ml/min.

7. What is pseudo about pseudotolerance?

Pseudotolerance is not a true tolerance to the pharmacologic effect of antihypertensive drugs. Rather, the term refers to retention of salt and water that occurs with certain antihypertensive classes (centrally acting sympatholytics, direct vasodilators, and α-adrenoreceptor antagonists) that ultimately blunts their antihypertensive effect. Addition of a diuretic to the regimen or an increase in the dose of the diuretic increases sodium excretion, reduces extracellular fluid volume (ECFV), and restores antihypertensive efficacy (see figure).

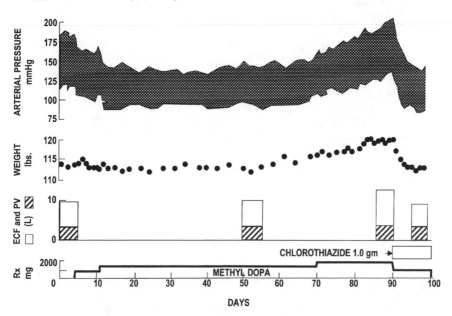

Typical response of arterial pressure, extracellular fluid (ECF) volume, plasma volume (PV) and weight to institution of a centrally acting sympatholytic (methyl dopa). Ultimately, salt and water retention increases weight, ECF volume, and PV with a consequent loss of blood pressure control, a phenomenon known as pseudotolerance. Addition of a diuretic (chlorothiazide) induces a natriuresis, decreases weight, ECF volume, and PV, and restores antihypertensive efficacy. (From Finnerty FA, Davidov M, Mroczek WJ, Gaurilovich L: Influence of extracellular fluid volume on response to antihypertensive drugs. Circ Res 27:I-71–I-80, 1970, with permission).

8. What drugs blunt the effect of antihypertensive agents?

- Nonsteroidal anti-inflammatory drugs
- Oral contraceptives
- Sympathomimetic amines
- Tricyclic antidepressants
- Appetite suppressants
- Cocaine and other illicit drugs
- Adrenal steroids
- Cyclosporine
- Erythropoietin

9. What causes pseudohypertension?

Pseudohypertension refers to measurement of spuriously high blood pressure due either to sclerotic brachial arteries in the elderly or to the use of a standard blood pressure cuff in patients with an arm circumference > 35 cm. In elderly hypertensive patients with significant vascular disease, atherosclerotic brachial arteries are poorly compressible and, hence, can result in falsely elevated blood pressures. Some, but not all, authorities suggest that palpation of the radial artery when the cuff is inflated above systolic blood pressure (i.e., Osler's maneuver) can identify this cause of pseudohypertension. Further, use of a large blood pressure cuff in all adult patients will minimize spurious hypertension and will not underestimate blood pressure in non-obese patients.

10. How do you document and manage office, or "white coat," hypertension?

Office hypertension can be a cause of apparently refractory hypertension. On the average, office blood pressures are 8 to 10 mmHg higher than home blood pressure determinations. Given the widespread availability of devices to monitor home blood pressure, most hypertensive patients should be encouraged to measure blood pressure at home. However, there are several caveats to home blood pressure monitoring. First, the patient should be instructed properly in the technique of measuring blood pressure. Second, the patient's cuff and technique must be validated in the physician's office. Third, hypertension at home is defined as blood pressures ≥ 135/85 mmHg. A significant disparity between office blood pressures and home blood pressure readings will readily identify the subset of patients with office hypertension, thereby avoiding unnecessary antihypertensive therapy. It is important to note that when there is a discrepancy between the two readings, electrocardiographic evidence of left ventricular hypertrophy correlates better with home blood pressure. An additional benefit to home blood pressure monitoring is that adjustments in drug therapy can logically be made on the basis of the log of home blood pressure determinations.

11. Name some common causes of secondary hypertension that can result in resistant hypertension.

Common Secondary Causes of Resistant Hypertension

DISEASE	CLUES TO DIAGNOSIS
Renal parenchymal disease	Proteinuria, hematuria, increased serum creatinine.
Renal artery stenosis	Age < 25 or > 60 at onset, abdominal bruit, peripheral vascular disease, sudden onset of difficult-to-control blood pressure in previously well-controlled patient.
Primary hyperaldosteronism	Unprovoked hypokalemia or potassium < 3.0 mEq/L in diuretic-treated patient.

(Table continued on next page.)

Common Secondary Causes of Resistant Hypertension (Continued)

DISEASE	CLUES TO DIAGNOSIS
Pheochromocytoma	Sweating, headache, palpitations.
Sleep apnea	Excessive snoring, daytime hyper-somnolence, interrupted sleep, obesity, polycythemia.

12. How do reactions to antihypertensive therapy cause resistant hypertension?

Secondary resistance to drug therapy can develop because of neurohumoral mechanisms induced by initial antihypertensive treatment. Stimulation of the sympathetic nervous system or the renin-angiotensin-aldosterone system, or both, results in fluid retention, increased cardiac output, and elevated peripheral resistance that can blunt the antihypertensive effect of diuretics or vasodilators. For example, in patients who develop compensatory hyperreninemia and increased circulating levels of angiotensin II during treatment with diuretics or vasodilators, the addition of an angiotensin-converting enzyme (ACE) inhibitor or β-blocker often restores control of blood pressure. Similarly, the tachycardia and elevated cardiac output induced by vasodilators can be ameliorated by a β-blocker or a centrally acting sympatholytic.

13. Construct a checklist for managing patients with resistant hypertension.

- Assess compliance with:
    - Medication regimen
    - Dietary salt restriction
- Is the antihypertensive regimen adequate?
- Are there any potential drug-induced causes?
- Does the patient have pseudohypertension?
- Does the patient have office hypertension?
- Have secondary causes been excluded?

14. From a practical perspective, assuming secondary causes of resistant hypertension have been excluded, how do you treat refractory hypertension?

Patient compliance with dietary salt restriction can be estimated from a 24-hour urine collection. Diuretic therapy should be optimized. Remember, an effective adjustment in the diuretic regimen will produce a 1–2 kg weight loss. Once an optimal diuretic regimen is achieved, additional antihypertensive agents may be required. If the patient is already receiving a diuretic, plus some combination of an ACE inhibitor (or angiotensin II antagonist), a calcium channel blocker, and β-blocker, make sure each of the drugs is titrated to its maximum dosage. If a fourth drug is required, a centrally acting sympatholytic (e.g., clonidine) is often effective. Although minoxidil is the most potent oral antihypertensive, its use is limited because of salt retention and hypertrichosis. With the large number of antihypertensive agents currently available, it is distinctly unusual to find a patient whose blood pressure cannot be normalized with a carefully designed four-drug regimen.

BIBLIOGRAPHY

1. Alderman MH, Budner N, Cohen H, et al: Prevalence of drug resistant hypertension. Hypertension 11:II-71–II-75, 1988.
2. Frohlich ED: Classification of resistant hypertension. Hypertension 11:II-67–II-70, 1988.

3. Gifford Jr, RW: An algorithm for the management of resistant hypertension. Hypertension 11:II-101–II-105, 1988.
4. Graves JW, Bloomfield RL, Buckalew Jr, VM: Plasma volume in resistant hypertension: Guide to pathophysiology and therapy. Am J Med Sci 298:361–365, 1989.
5. Joint National Committee on Prevention, Detection, Evaluation, and Treatment of High Blood Pressure: The Sixth Report of the Joint National Committee on Prevention, Detection, Evaluation, and Treatment of High Blood Pressure (JNC VI). Arch Intern Med 157:2413–2445, 1997.
6. Linfors EW, Feussner JR, Blessing CL, et al: Spurious hypertension in the obese patient. Effect of sphygmomanometer cuff size on prevalence of hypertension. Arch Intern Med 144:1482–1485, 1984.
7. Setaro JF, Black HR: Refractory hypertension. N Engl J Med 327:543–547, 1992.
8. Yakovlevitch M, Black HR: Resistant hypertension in a tertiary care clinic. Arch Intern Med 151:1786–1792, 1991.

19. HYPERTENSION IN PATIENTS WITH DIABETES MELLITUS

Mahboob Rahman, M.D., M.S.

1. Are diabetic patients at high risk for cardiovascular disease?

Yes. The risk of having a cardiovascular event in a diabetic patient is as high as a nondiabetic patient who already has had a myocardial infarction.

2. Why are diabetic patients at high risk for cardiovascular disease?

This is probably due to the presence of multiple risk factors for **atherosclerosis**, such as hypertension, obesity, and hyperlipidemia. Endothelial dysfunction may predispose to the development and progression of atherosclerotic lesions.

3. Why is control of hypertension so important in diabetic patients?

1. High blood pressure (BP) is associated with worsening of all manifestations of diabetic end-organ damage, including nephropathy, retinopathy, and neuropathy.

2. Aggressive control of BP has been shown to slow the progression of these conditions.

3. High BP and diabetes mellitus are independent risk factors for vascular disease; the coexistence of both puts a patient at much higher risk for atherosclerosis.

4. What pathophysiologic factors contribute to the development of hypertension in diabetic patients?

1. High levels of insulin (in patients with type 2 diabetes mellitus) may increase sympathetic nervous system activity, promote renal sodium retention, and increase systemic BP.

2. Filtered glucose is reabsorbed by the proximal tubule by a sodium-glucose transporter, resulting in a parallel rise in sodium reabsorption.

3. In patients with type 1 diabetes mellitus, the development of hypertension is associated closely with the development and progression of diabetic nephropathy.

5. List some clinical features of hypertension in diabetic patients.

Orthostatic hypotension: Patients with long-standing diabetes frequently have associated autonomic neuropathy. This may result in a significant decline in BP in the upright position. It is important to measure BP in the seated and standing positions in diabetic patients.

Salt sensitivity: Because sodium retention is one of the mechanisms mediating the development of hypertension in diabetic patients, BP frequently is salt sensitive and is lowered by restriction of dietary sodium intake.

Nondipping profile on ambulatory BP monitoring: Many patients with essential hypertension have a decline in BP at night, which is usually referred to as the nocturnal dip. This decline in BP often is blunted or absent in diabetic patients. The sustained hypertension resulting from the absence of a nocturnal dip may contribute to the increased severity of target organ damage seen in these patients.

White coat hypertension: This phenomenon is common diabetic patients. It is helpful to obtain BP readings outside the physician's office.

6. What level of BP control should you aim for in diabetic patients?

< 130/80 mm Hg. Even lower levels of BP are desirable in diabetic patients with evidence of diabetic nephropathy.

7. How is the target BP different from what you would aim for in other patients and why?

In most patients with essential hypertension, current guidelines recommend that the BP goal should be < 140/90 mm Hg; however, it has been shown that diabetic patients benefit in terms of reduction of cardiovascular events and slowing progression of renal disease by reducing BP to even lower levels.

8. List lifestyle modifications that you would advise to the diabetic hypertensive patient.
 • Weight control through diet and regular exercise
 • Restriction of dietary sodium intake
 • Cessation of smoking

9. Why is weight control important in the diabetic hypertensive patient?

Approximately 85% of patients with type 2 diabetes are obese. If patients can maintain a weight at or close to their ideal body weight, **insulin resistance improves**, and glycemic control and BP may be controlled better with fewer medications.

10. What is the significance of proteinuria in the hypertensive diabetic patient?

The presence of proteinuria generally indicates the presence of **diabetic nephropathy**. In early stages, protein in the urine may not be detected by a dipstick urinalysis. Even a small quantity of protein excretion (**microalbuminuria**, consisting of urinary albumin excretion of 30–300 mg/day) is associated with progression of diabetic nephropathy and predicts the development of cardiovascular disease.

11. How would the presence of proteinuria change the management of the hypertensive diabetic patient?

Patients who have > 1 g of protein excretion per day are at particularly high risk for progression of renal insufficiency and benefit the most by aggressive BP control to < 125/75 mm Hg.

12. What is the role of angiotensin-converting enzyme (ACE) inhibitors and angiotensin receptor blockers in the management of hypertension in diabetic patients?

Use of ACE inhibitors or angiotensin receptor blockers has been shown to reduce proteinuria and slow down the rate of decline of renal function in patients with type 1 diabetes and nephropathy as well as patients with the more common type 2 diabetes. ACE inhibitors may be superior to conventional antihypertensive drug therapy in reducing the incidence of cardiovascular events; however, the results of ongoing large studies are awaited to confirm this hypothesis.

13. Which is more important for the diabetic patient with renal disease: BP lowering or inhibition of angiotensin?

The inhibition of angiotensin achieved with either ACE inhibitors or angiotensin receptor blockers provides more protection against the progression of renal failure than that achieved by lowering BP to a comparable degree with other classes of medications.

14. Are diuretics effective in treatment of hypertension in diabetic patients?

Yes. Diuretics have been shown to reduce the risk of stroke and cardiovascular end points. There may be a slight rise in blood glucose at high doses of thiazide diuretics; this usually can be controlled with modification of antidiabetic therapy.

15. What is the role of combination therapy in the management of hypertension in diabetic patients?

Many patients require more than one antihypertensive drug to obtain target BP. The use of combination drugs (such as ACE inhibitors plus diuretics) reduces the number of pills a patient has to take and takes advantage of synergistic effect of these agents on BP.

16. Show a systematic approach for optimizing the antihypertensive drug regimen in the management of hypertension in diabetic patients.

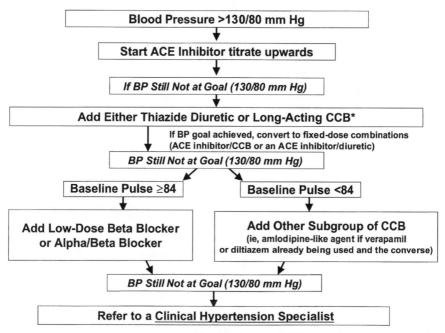

Algorithm for achieving target BP goals in hypertension in diabetic patients. DHP = dihydropyridines. (Modified from Bakris GL, Williams M, Dworkin L, et al: Preserving renal function in adults with hypertension and diabetes: A consensus approach. National Kidney Foundation Hypertension and Diabetes Executive Committees Working Group. Am J Kidney Dis 36(3):646–661, 2000.)

BIBLIOGRAPHY

1. Bakris GL, Williams M, Dworkin L, et al: Preserving renal function in adults with hypertension and diabetes: A consensus approach. National Kidney Foundation Hypertension and Diabetes Executive Committees Working Group. Am J Kidney Dis 36:646–661, 2000.
2. Cooper ME, Johnston CI: Optimizing treatment of hypertension in patients with diabetes. JAMA 283:3177–3179, 2000.
3. Deedwania PC: Hypertension and diabetes: New therapeutic options. Arch Intern Med 160:1585–1594, 2000.

20. ISOLATED SYSTOLIC HYPERTENSION AND HYPERTENSION IN THE ELDERLY

Patrick S. T. Hayden, M.D.

1. Define isolated systolic hypertension (ISH).
Systolic blood pressure (BP) ≥ 160 mm Hg and diastolic BP < 90 mm Hg.

2. In which age group is ISH prevalent?
The elderly.

3. What is the significance of the prevalence of ISH in the elderly?
The U.S. population is aging, with estimates that 75 million people will be ≥ 65 years old by 2040.

4. How common is ISH?
ISH is one of the most prevalent forms of hypertension, present in two thirds of hypertensive people > 60 years old.

5. Why is ISH common in the elderly?
Control rates for BP are lowest in the elderly, primarily because of inadequate aggressiveness and attention to elevated systolic BPs. For patients ≥ 70 years old, only 25% of African-Americans and 18% of whites have acceptable BP control.

6. What about the old adage that one's age plus 100 reflects an acceptable systolic BP?
The old adage is no longer acceptable. Framingham data show that for men aged 55 to 74, all-cause mortality more than doubled in those with ISH compared with normotensive controls. The Systolic Hypertension in Elderly Program (SHEP) study reveals that decreasing the systolic BP in older individuals with ISH reduced morbidity and mortality, as individuals with ISH are at increased risk for stroke, myocardial infarction, other cardiovascular disease, and death.

7. Describe the relationship between BP and age.
In Western industrialized societies, systolic BP increases with age; diastolic blood pressure increases as well but only until age 55, at which time it usually declines (see figure, next page).

8. Explain the pathophysiology for age-related changes in BP.
The rising systolic BP that occurs with aging reflects an elevation in **peripheral vascular resistance** resulting from stiffness of large arteries that occurs as individuals grow older. Diastolic BP also increases as peripheral vascular resistance rises; however, progressive stiffening of large arteries lowers diastolic BP. Stiffening of blood vessels with advancing age results in a gradual increase in **pulse pressure** (i.e., the difference between systolic and diastolic pressure).

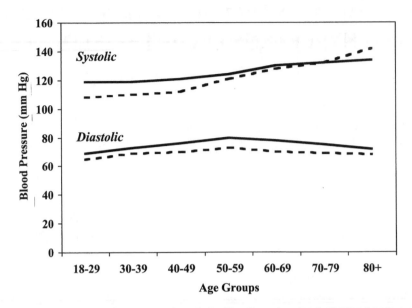

Relationship between blood pressure and age in healthy Caucasian men (*solid lines*) and women (*dashed lines*.)

9. Why do arteries stiffen with age?

In the walls of large arteries, elastin is replaced by collagen, resulting in decreased compliance. This process, arteriosclerosis, causes dilation and lengthening of the large arteries, such as the aorta and its branches, as fibrosis and hypertrophy of the arterial muscularis occur. Hypertension accelerates arteriosclerosis, and a vicious cycle ensues.

10. Are atherosclerosis and arteriosclerosis synonymous?

No. **Atherosclerosis** refers to the process of abnormal cholesterol deposition in the inner layers of arteries.

11. Is the pulse pressure an independent predictor of morbidity?

Yes. Pulse pressure is an independent predictor of **congestive heart failure**. For each 10-mm Hg increase in pulse pressure, one's risk for congestive heart failure increases by 14%.

12. Which predicts cardiovascular risk more precisely, systolic or diastolic BP?

Systolic BP.

13. Does antihypertensive therapy ameliorate this risk?

Yes. The SHEP study showed that BP-lowering therapy significantly decreased the risk of **stroke**, whether fatal or nonfatal, in people ≥ 60 years old with ISH. Total stroke incidence was decreased by 36% in the active treatment group; nonfatal myocardial infarction and coronary death had a 27% lower incidence rate versus placebo; and for all causes of death, the active treatment group had a 13% lower death rate versus placebo.

14. When treating ISH, what is the target BP?

Particularly if a patient has diabetes or congestive heart failure, a BP of no greater than 130/85 mm Hg is desirable.

15. Should ISH be treated in the old elderly (aged 70–84)?

Yes, according to data from the Swedish Trial in Old Patients with Hypertension (STOP-Hypertension). These individuals experienced significant reductions in morbidity and mortality related to stroke and myocardial infarction.

16. What about adjunctive therapy?

Lifestyle changes—weight loss, salt and dietary restriction, and exercise—play an important role.

17. Discuss agents that should be used with caution in ISH.

β-Blockers. The JNC in 1997 no longer recommended β-blockers for first-line treatment for ISH because data reveal that BP control rates are meager compared with rates achieved with diuretics. The deleterious effect of β-blockers on cardiac output coupled with their high rate of side effects render this class of antihypertensives problematic in the elderly individual with ISH.

Thiazides. A post-hoc analysis of the SHEP study showed that hypokalemia, even in the presence of diuretic-induced normotension, negated the beneficial effect of BP control achieved with the use of thiazides. For individuals rendered normotensive but hypokalemic, the risk of stroke and coronary artery disease was similar to those with hypertension. Thiazides should be used for the treatment of ISH only if associated hypokalemia is monitored and corrected.

18. Who fares better in terms of cardiovascular risk: the older individual with elevated systolic BP and diastolic BP or the individual with ISH?

The older individual with elevated systolic BP and diastolic BP has less morbidity and mortality:

1. Coronary heart disease is inversely related to diastolic BP at any systolic BP ≥ 120 mm Hg.

2. There is an association between malnutrition or malignancy and low diastolic BP.

3. Decreased diastolic BP translates to decreased coronary artery flow, predisposing to ischemia.

CONTROVERSY

19. Do all medicine regimens confer fairly equal benefit in the treatment of ISH?

The Joint National Committee (JNC) VI recommends a **diuretic** and **calcium channel blocker** as therapy of choice because data abound suggesting decreased rates of myocardial infarction, heart failure, and stroke. SHEP and the Systolic Hypertension in Europe trial support the use of thiazides with or without β-blockers and long-acting calcium channel blockers when treating ISH. Angiotensin-converting enzyme inhibitors are effective in older individuals, particularly those with congestive heart failure.

BIBLIOGRAPHY

1. Applegate WB, et al: Nonpharmacologic intervention to reduce BP in older patients with mild hypertension. Arch Intern Med 152:1162–1166, 1992.
2. Dahlöf B, et al: Morbidity and mortality in the Swedish Trial in Old Patients with Hypertension (STOP-Hypertension). Lancet 338:1281–1285, 1991.
3. Franklin SS, et al: Is pulse pressure useful in predicting risk for coronary heart disease? The Framingham Heart Study. Circulation 100:354–360, 1999.
4. Franse LV, et al: Hypokalemia associated with diuretic use and cardiovascular events in the Systolic Hypertension in the Elderly Program. Hypertension 35:1025–1030, 2000.
5. Insua JT, et al: Drug treatment of hypertension in the elderly: A meta-analysis. Ann Intern Med 121:355–362, 1994.
6. Izzo JL, et al: Importance of systolic BP in older Americans. Hypertension 35:1021–1024, 2000.
7. Messerli FH, et al: Are β-blockers efficacious as first-line therapy for hypertension in the elderly? A systematic review. JAMA 279:1903–1907, 1998.
8. Ostfeld AM, Havlik RJ, Guralnik L: Epidemiology and treatment of hypertension in older persons. In Laragh JH, Brenner BM (eds): Hypertension: Pathophysiology, Diagnosis and Management, 2nd ed. New York, Raven Press, 1995.
9. SHEP Cooperative Research Group: Prevention of stroke by antihypertensive drug treatment in older persons with isolated systolic hypertension: Final results of the systolic hypertension in the elderly program (SHEP). JAMA 265:3255–3264, 1991.
10. Staessen JA, et al: Risks of untreated and treated isolated systolic hypertension in the elderly: Meta-analysis of outcome trials. Lancet 355:865–872, 2000.

21. NON-DRUG THERAPY OF HYPERTENSION

Robert L. Haynie, M.D., Ph.D., and Jackson T. Wright, Jr., M.D., Ph.D.

1. What is the role of non-drug therapies in the management of hypertension?

- Non-drug therapies have the potential to:
  Lower blood pressure
  Prevent the development of hypertension
  Reduce other cardiovascular risk factors
- Modalities consistently shown to be effective are summarized in the table below and include weight loss, sodium restriction, limitation of alcohol intake, and institution of a diet high in fruits, vegetables, fiber, and low-fat dairy products (i.e., the Dietary Approaches to Stop Hypertension [DASH] study diet).
- While diets high in calcium and potassium have consistently shown efficacy in lowering blood pressure, supplementing diet with these cations has shown limited clinical benefit.
- Aerobic exercise is required for weight reduction/control and it reduces cardiovascular risk. However, its independent effect on lowering blood pressure is uncertain.

Non-Drug Antihypertensive Therapy

COMPELLING EVIDENCE SUPPORTING	SUGGESTIVE EVIDENCE TO SUPPORT	CARDIOVASCULAR RISK REDUCTION
Weight reduction	↑ Dietary potassium	↓ Saturated fat
Salt restriction	↑ Dietary calcium	↓ Cholesterol
DASH diet	Aerobic exercise	Avoid tobacco
Alcohol moderation		Aerobic exercise

2. What data suggest that weight reduction ameliorates hypertension?

- Current guidelines define overweight as a body mass index (BMI) > 25 kg/m^2 and obesity as a BMI > 30 kg/m^2 (see table, top of next page).
- According to the latest NHANES survey, 55% of US adults over age 20 are overweight or obese.
- BMI > 27 kg/m^2 or increased waist circumference (> 34 inches in women or > 39 inches in men) is linked to a higher prevalence of hypertension, and hypertension prevalence doubles with obesity (BMI > 30 kg/m^2).
- Weight loss of as little as 10 lbs will significantly lower blood pressure.
- In many patients, the first goal may be to prevent further weight gain in hypertensives who show continuing weight gain.
- Weight reduction and control require both calorie restriction and increase in activity level.
- Recidivism is to be expected and can frustrate both patient and provider.

Classifications for BMI

WEIGHT	BMI
Underweight	< 18.5
Normal weight	18.5–24.9 kg/m^2
Overweight	25–29.9 kg/m^2
Obesity	> 35 kg/m^2
Extreme obesity	≥ 40 kg/m^2

3. What strategies are useful in weight reduction and control?

- In overweight (BMI > 25 kg/m^2) or obese (BMI > 30 kg/m^2) hypertensives, the initial goal is loss of 10% body weight over six months at a rate of 1–2 lbs/wk.
- Weight loss requires reduction in calories, as well as a decrease in dietary fat.
- Dietary referral should be considered with the goal of reducing current caloric intake by 500–1000 kcal/day.
- An effective strategy must include a program of increased daily activity (e.g., stairs vs. elevators, walking rather than riding) as well as an appropriate, regular exercise regimen on **most** days of week.
- Very cautious use of weight loss drugs may be considered as part of an overall program in patients with BMI > 30 kg/m^2. Sibutramine (Meridia) can substantially elevate blood pressure and is contraindicated in hypertensives.
- Weight loss surgery may be considered for patients who have failed other measures and with BMI > 40 kg/m^2 (BMI > 35 kg/m^2 if obesity-related comorbid conditions are present).

4. What is the effect of dietary sodium on blood pressure and the prevalence of hypertension?

- Current average U.S. sodium consumption is approximately 150 mmol/day.
- The evidence relating salt intake to elevated blood pressure is compelling.
    - Inter-population studies suggest a 6–8-fold increase in hypertension prevalence in societies with high vs. low dietary sodium.
    - Multiple segments of the U.S. population experience an increase in blood pressure with increased salt ingestion.
    - Approximately half of all hypertensives are salt-sensitive. Hypertensives most likely to be salt-sensitive include diabetics, the elderly, obese hypertensives, and those with concomitant kidney disease.
- Black hypertensives reportedly have a higher incidence of salt-sensitivity. but many of these reports may reflect a higher prevalence of associated risk factors for salt-sensitivity.
- In addition to its effect on raising blood pressure, several studies associate high sodium intake with evidence of target organ damage (i.e., left ventricular hypertrophy, proteinuria).
- The effect of sodium restriction on blood pressure has been shown to be additive to other dietary changes.
- The goal is to reduce sodium intake to < 100 mmol/day (equivalent to approximately 6 grams salt or 2.4 grams sodium) (see table, next page).

- Multiple studies confirm that sodium intake to the recommended levels (60–100 mmol/day) is safe and effective in reducing blood pressure. Moreover, this level of sodium restriction decreases the risk of hypokalemia in hypertensives on diuretics and induces regression of left ventricular hypertrophy.
- Achieving this salt intake goal will require teaching the patient to read food labels as well as the usual advice on decreasing discretionary use.

Usual vs. Goal Sodium Intake

	US AVG. CONSUMPTION/DAY	GOAL
Sodium (mmol/day)	150	< 100
Salt (grams/day)	9	< 6
Sodium (grams/day)	3.6	< 2.4

5. What is the role of alcohol in the hypertensive patient?
- More than two drinks per day of alcohol is associated with higher blood pressure and an increased prevalence of hypertension. In a large HMO study, > 6 drinks/day doubled the prevalence of a blood pressure >160/95 mmHg.
- Not surprisingly, adherence to antihypertensive treatment is also impaired with excessive alcohol intake.
- It is worth noting that abrupt withdrawal after a binge may substantially elevate blood pressure for up to three days, and may complicate the assessment of adequacy of antihypertensive regimen if clinic visits occur during this interval.
- A detailed history of alcohol consumption should be obtained and patients counseled to reduce intake to < 24 oz of beer, 10 oz of wine, or 2 oz of 100 proof spirits. (Amount should be reduced by ½ in women.)

6. Are dietary strategies that do not alter salt or caloric intake effective in reducing blood pressure?
- A diet that is high in fruits, vegetables, grains, nuts, and low-fat dairy products with smaller amounts of red meat, fish and poultry (DASH diet) was shown to reduce blood pressure by 5/3 mmHg compared to the usual U.S. diet even without salt restriction or caloric reduction.
- Sodium restriction from the average 145 mmol/day to 67 mmol/day produced additional 3/1.5 mmHg decrease in blood pressure.
- The results of these dietary manipulations are exaggerated in African Americans and women.
- However, the effects of dietary manipulations are seen in both men and women, African Americans and other races, and in both hypertensives and normotensives.
- These reductions in blood pressure are comparable to monotherapy with most antihypertensive drug classes. In normotensives, the DASH diet may significantly slow or prevent the progression to hypertension.

7. How should the control of other cardiovascular risk factors influence the care of the hypertensive patient?
- It is important to keep in mind that hypertension is one risk factor in a patient population that typically has several cardiovascular risk factors.

- Careful identification, assessment, and treatment of all risk factors are critical in order to reduce cardiovascular morbidity and mortality.

BIBLIOGRAPHY

1. Appel LJ, Moore TJ, Obarzanek E, et al, and the DASH Collaborative Research Group. A clinical trial of the effects of dietary patterns on blood pressure. N Engl J Med 336:1117–1124, 1997.
2. National High Blood Pressure Education Program: National High Blood Pressure Education Program Working Group Report on Primary Prevention of Hypertension. Arch Intern Med 153:186–208, 1993.
3. The Practical Guide. Identification, Evaluation, and Treatment of Overweight and Obesity in Adults. Bethesda, MD, NIH/NHLBI, 2000, NIH publication no 00-4084.
4. Sacks FM, Svetkey LP, Vollmer WM, et al: Effects on blood pressure of reduced dietary sodium and the dietary approaches to stop hypertension (DASH) diet. DASH-Sodium Collaborative Research Group. N Engl J Med 344:3–10, 2001.
5. Whelton P K, Appel LJ, Espeland MA, et al: Sodium reduction and weight loss in the treatment of hypertension in older persons: A randomized controlled trial of nonpharmacologic interventions in the elderly (TONE). TONE Collaborative Research Group. JAMA 279:839–846, 1998.

22. TREATMENT OF HYPERTENSIVE CRISES

Donald E. Hricik, M.D.

1. What is a hypertensive crisis?

A syndrome of acute, severe hypertension characterized either as:
- A **hypertensive urgency**, in which there is no associated end-organ damage or
- A **hypertensive emergency**, in which there is associated end-organ damage

2. What is the goal of management of patients with hypertensive urgencies?

To lower blood pressure (BP) within 24 hours, usually with oral agents.

3. Is there any advantage to using an agent that lowers BP more rapidly?

No. There are no data to suggest that more rapid lowering of BP is beneficial, whereas some data suggest that overly aggressive reduction of BP in this setting may be harmful. Immediate-release nifedipine—previously a popular drug in this setting—now is probably contraindicated because of the tendency for this agent to cause precipitous hypotension.

4. List the drugs and doses favored for the treatment of hypertensive urgencies.

Oral Agents for the Treatment of Hypertensive Urgencies

DRUG	DOSE
Clonidine	0.1–0.2 mg orally; repeat hourly as required
Labetalol	200–400 mg orally; repeat every 2–3 h
Captopril	25 mg orally; repeat every 4–6 h
Prazosin	1–2 mg orally; repeat hourly

5. Define hypertensive encephalopathy.

A syndrome of cerebrovascular dysfunction and neurologic impairment associated with severe hypertension. It is one of the life-threatening forms of end-organ damage that can occur in patients with hypertensive emergencies. Clinical manifestations include headache, restlessness, nausea, vomiting, confusion, and seizures. Reduction in BP usually produces rapid clinical improvement. The diagnosis may be in doubt until neurologic improvement occurs after systemic BP is reduced.

6. Describe the pathophysiology of hypertensive encephalopathy.

Under normal circumstances, cerebral arterioles constrict in response to an acute rise in BP, a form of **autoregulation** designed to prevent an increase in blood flow during periods of increased BP. In patients with severe hypertension, the autoregulatory capacity of such vessels may be exceeded, leading to cerebral vasodilation. This vasodilation leads to disruption of the blood-brain barrier, focal areas of cerebral edema, and localized changes in the flux of ions and neurotransmitters that impair neuronal function.

7. Discuss the principles underlying management of patients with hypertensive emergencies.

Management requires hospitalization, most often in an **intensive care unit**. The goal of initial treatment is to reduce BP, but not necessarily to normal levels. Autoregulatory mechanisms in the brain, heart, and kidney usually protect these organs from ischemia when BP is decreased suddenly. In patients with severe hypertension, the lower limit of autoregulation may be shifted upward so that autoregulation fails at higher levels of pressure, increasing the risk of organ hypoperfusion when BP is suddenly decreased to *normal* levels.

8. Specifically, what is the initial goal of therapy?

To reduce mean arterial BP by approximately 25% within 2 to 3 hours, or to a BP of about 160/100 mm Hg. More rapid reduction of BP may be warranted in patients with aortic dissection or acute pulmonary edema.

9. List desirable features for drugs used to treat hypertensive emergencies.
- Rapid onset of action and rapid reversibility
- Reduction of total peripheral resistance without a decrease in cardiac output
- No central nervous system side effects (i.e., sedation) that might be confused with hypertensive encephalopathy
- Steep dose-response curve
- Low toxic-to-therapeutic ratio

10. What drugs are favored for the treatment of hypertensive emergencies?

In general, hypertensive emergencies are associated with severe vasoconstriction. Therefore, vasodilators are the preferred initial agents for hypertensive emergencies.

11. What drugs are not recommended?

Diuretics, unless the patient exhibits signs of pulmonary edema.

12. List the drugs most often used for the treatment of hypertensive emergencies.

Parenteral Agents for the Treatment of Hypertensive Emergencies

DRUG	DOSE	ONSET OF ACTION	COMMENTS
Nitroprusside	0.25–10 µg/kg/min IV infusion	30 sec–1 min	Drug of choice for hypertensive encephalopathy, left ventricular failure with pulmonary edema, aortic dissection. Prolonged use can cause thiocyanate intoxication
Nitroglycerin	5–100 µg/min IV infusion	1–3 min	Drug of choice for unstable angina or myocardial infarction. May cause headache, tachycardia
Labetalol	20–80 mg IV bolus q 10 min or 2 mg/min IV infusion	5–10 min	May cause nausea. Avoid in asthma congestive heart failure, or third-degree heart block
Hydralazine	5–10 mg IV or IM q 20 min	10–20 min	Drug of choice for severe eclampsia. Avoid in coronary artery disease. May cause headache, tachycardia

Table continued on next page.

Parenteral Agents for the Treatment of Hypertensive Emergencies (Continued)

DRUG	DOSE	ONSET OF ACTION	COMMENTS
Enalaprilat	0.625–1.25 mg IV every 6 h	15 min	May cause renal failure in patients with bilateral renal artery stenosis
Fenoldopam	0.1–0.6 μg/kg/min	15–20 min	May cause headache, nausea, flushing. Natriuretic

IV = intravenous; IM = intramuscular; q = every.

BIBLIOGRAPHY

1. Gales MA: Oral antihypertensives for hypertensive urgencies. Ann Pharmacother 28:352–358, 1994.
2. Gifford RW: Management of hypertensive crises. JAMA 266:829–835, 1991.
3. Healton EB, Brust JC, Feinfeld DA, Thomson GE: Hypertensive encephalopathy and the neurologic manifestations of malignant hypertension. Neurology 32:127–132, 1982.
4. Kitiyakara C, Guzman NJ: Malignant hypertension and hypertensive emergencies. J Am Soc Nephrol 9:133–142, 1998.

23. DIURETICS

Lavinia Negrea, M.D.

1. List the long-term benefits of diuretics in treating mild-to-moderate hypertension.
1. Reduction in cerebrovascular morbidity and mortality
2. Reduction in cardiovascular morbidity and mortality
3. Regression of left ventricular hypertrophy
4. Prevention of the development of congestive heart failure

2. What are the concerns with use of diuretics in treating hypertension?
Individual trials usually have not shown a significant effect on coronary heart disease mortality. The reasons for this are unclear but might be related to the relatively short duration of many trials, to adverse diuretic-induced metabolic effects (e.g., hyperlipidemia, hypokalemia), or to the fact that hypertension is not as great a risk factor for coronary heart disease as it is for cerebrovascular disease.

3. What diuretic classes are commonly used to treat hypertension?
Thiazides (mainstay of treatment in patients with essential hypertension and normal renal function)
Loop diuretics
Potassium-sparing diuretics

4. Give examples of diuretics and dosing guidelines used in the treatment of hypertension.

GENERIC NAME (TRADE NAME)	DOSING INTERVAL*	DOSE RANGE (mg)[†]
Thiazides		
Chlorothiazide (Diuril)	qd or bid	125–500
Chlorthalidone (Hygroton)	qd	12.5–50
Hydrochlorothiazide (HydroDIURIL)	qd	12.5–50
Indapamide (Lozol)	qd	2.5–5.0
Metolazone (Zaroxolyn)	qd	2.5–5.0
Loop diuretics		
Bumetanide (Bumex)	qd or bid	0.5–5.0
Ethacrynic acid (Edecrin)	qd or bid	25–100
Furosemide (Lasix)	qd or bid	20–320
Torsemide (Demadex)	qd or bid	5–200
Potassium-sparing diuretics		
Amiloride (Midamor)	qd or bid	5–10
Spironolactone (aldactone)	qd or bid	25–100
Triamterene (Dyrenium)	qd or bid	50–150

* To encourage adherence, drugs that have a qd dosing regimen are recommended.
[†] Dosages should be individualized by titration of antihypertensive effect.
qd = every day; bid = twice a day.

5. How do thiazide diuretics reduce blood pressure (BP)?

Thiazide diuretics inhibit sodium and chloride reabsorption in the distal convoluted tubule, where 5% to 8% of the filtered sodium is reabsorbed. Plasma and extracellular fluid volume consequently decrease, and the cardiac output decreases. With long-term use, plasma volume returns partially toward normal, but at the same time, total peripheral resistance decreases (see figure). The long-term hemodynamic profile shows a decrease in BP, a normal cardiac output, and a reduced total peripheral resistance. The factors responsible for the secondary vasodilation are unclear but might be related to a decrease in the sodium and calcium content of vascular smooth muscle.

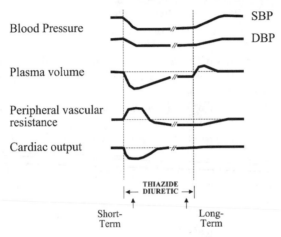

Hemodynamic profile during short-term and long-term diuretic therapy in essential hypertension. SBP = systolic blood pressure; DBP = diastolic blood pressure.

6. Are there any patient populations that respond better to diuretics than to other classes of antihypertensive drugs?

Elderly and African-American patients. Hypertensive patients who respond to diuretics are generally **salt-sensitive** and exhibit a decreased plasma renin activity compared with nonresponders. There is significant overlap between the two groups, however.

7. Discuss the role of diuretics in combination therapy for hypertension.

Diuretics are useful in combination with all other classes of antihypertensive agents and produce an added reduction in BP. They are particularly effective in combination with **angiotensin-converting enzyme (ACE) inhibitors or angiotensin II receptor blockers (ARBs)**. Certain drug classes (i.e., α-blockers, direct vasodilators) require a diuretic in the antihypertensive regimen to prevent the development of salt and water retention, which ultimately attenuates the initial antihypertensive effect.

8. What are some of the common reasons for resistance to the antihypertensive action of diuretics?

1. **Lack of dietary sodium restriction.** Because long-term diuretic administration stimulates the renin-angiotensin-aldosterone system, with consequent salt

retention, **excessive dietary sodium** intake can nullify the diuretic's ability to maintain a volume-contracted state.

2. **Ingestion of nonsteroidal anti-inflammatory drugs (NSAIDs).** Most NSAIDs blunt the effect of diuretics; this is partly due to altering the renal hemodynamics through inhibition of prostaglandin synthesis.

3. **Renal insufficiency.** Progressive **renal dysfunction** limits the renal response to diuretics. Thiazide diuretics are generally ineffective at creatinine clearance values of < 30 ml/min.

9. Discuss electrolyte and acid-base abnormalities that are associated with thiazide diuretic use.

Hypokalemia is dose related and worse with long-acting agents. Sodium reabsorption in the distal convoluted tubule and in cortical collecting duct favors potassium secretion. By increasing sodium delivery in this region, thiazide and loop-blocking diuretics are kaliuretic. Hypokalemia can blunt the hypotensive response to diuretic therapy and predispose to ventricular arrhythmias in patients receiving digoxin or in patients with ischemic heart disease.

Hyperkalemia occurs in patients given potassium-sparing diuretics alone or in combination with potassium supplements to treat or prevent hypokalemia. Risk factors for hyperkalemia in patients receiving potassium-sparing diuretics include renal insufficiency, hyporeninemic hypoaldosteronism (type IV renal tubular acidosis), and drugs that limit potassium excretion (e.g., NSAIDs, ACE inhibitors, cyclosporine, trimethoprim).

Hyponatremia is reported more commonly with thiazide diuretics than other classes. The postulated mechanisms responsible for thiazide-induced hyponatremia include volume depletion resulting in enhanced secretion of antidiuretic hormone, inhibition of sodium chloride cotransport in the distal tubule leading to inability to dilute urine maximally, and resetting of the osmostat. Older women who are leaner than gender-matched and age-matched controls are at increased risk to develop thiazide-induced hyponatremia. Predisposition to this complication is long-lasting.

Hypercalcemia occurs secondary to stimulation of calcium reabsorption in the distal tubule by thiazide diuretics. It is usually subclinical.

Hyperuricemia occurs because diuretics increase reabsorption and blunt secretion of urate in the nephron. Gout develops only infrequently.

Metabolic alkalosis occurs as a result of volume depletion (**contraction alkalosis**) and development of secondary hyperaldosteronism. The latter stimulates distal proton secretion.

10. When are loop diuretics preferred over thiazides in treating BP?

Loop-blocking diuretics generally are indicated in hypertensive patients with creatinine clearance values <30 ml/min. As renal failure progresses, endogenous organic acids accumulate and compete with diuretics in the proximal tubule for transport into the tubular lumen, making thiazide diuretics less effective at the usual doses. A logical increase in the dose is associated with increased side effects. In patients with renal insufficiency, salt retention plays a major role in the elevation of BP, and more natriuresis is needed. Loop diuretics block sodium chloride reabsorption in the thick ascending limb of the loop of Henle, a site where 25% to 40% of sodium is reabsorbed. When the effect of the diuretic subsides, urinary sodium excretion decreases below control levels. This **diuretic rebound** is mediated by the activation of the renin-angiotensin-aldosterone system. Short-acting loop diuretics require more than once-daily dosing to be effective in hypertensive patients with renal insufficiency and avid salt retention.

11. When is spironolactone indicated?

Spironolactone competitively inhibits the binding of aldosterone to the mineralocorticoid receptor in the collecting tubule and is specific medical therapy for hypertension in primary aldosteronism. Data suggest that spironolactone reduces cardiovascular morbidity and mortality in patients with systolic dysfunction. Consequently, it is a useful adjunctive agent in the subset of hypertensive patients with systolic dysfunction and New York Heart Association class III or IV heart failure.

12. What is the clinical utility of potassium-sparing diuretics in essential hypertension?

Potassium-sparing diuretics have weak natriuretic activity, leading to excretion of only 1% to 2% of filtered sodium, and seldom are used as initial therapy for essential hypertension. They are used, however, in combination with thiazide diuretics to enhance the natriuretic effect of the latter, while minimizing their kaliuretic effect.

13. List common combinations that include potassium-sparing diuretics.

Hydrochlorothiazide (HCTZ) and a potassium-sparing diuretic are common combinations:

Maxzide and Dyazide (HCTZ and triamterene)
Moduretic (HCTZ and amiloride)
Aldactazide (HCTZ and spironolactone)

CONTROVERSY

14. Describe cardiovascular complications that have been associated with thiazide diuretic use.

Ventricular arrhythmias. Whether diuretic therapy increases the risk of arrhythmias is controversial. Hypokalemia rather than a direct diuretic effect is responsible for any proarrhythmic effect, which is probably confined to high-risk groups.

Hypercholesterolemia. Total cholesterol and low-density lipoprotein cholesterol reportedly have been increased by 6.5% and 15% in short-term studies; however, this has not been verified in long-term trials. Evidence suggests that these effects on lipids do not occur when low doses of thiazides are used.

Glucose intolerance. Fasting glucose levels increased 3.2 mg/dl after 5 years in young patients treated with diuretics but were similar to increments in the placebo group. In contrast, elderly patients experienced an increase of 6.5 mg/dl, a value significantly greater than the placebo group. Thiazide diuretics can decrease glucose tolerance, but they rarely cause diabetes.

BIBLIOGRAPHY

1. Brater DC: Diuretic therapy. N Engl J Med 339:387–395, 1998.
2. Greenberg A: Diuretic complications. Am J Med Sci 319:10–24, 2000.
3. Joint National Committee on Prevention, Detection, Evaluation, and Treatment of High Blood Pressure: The sixth report of the Joint National Committee on Prevention, Detection, Evaluation, and Treatment of High Blood Pressure. Arch Intern Med 157:2413–2445, 1997.
4. Kaplan NM: Diuretics: Correct use in hypertension. Semin Nephrol 19:569–574, 1999.
5. Puschett JB: Diuretics and the therapy of hypertension. Am J Med Sci 319:1–9, 2000.
6. Valvo E, D'Angelo A, Maschio G: Diuretics in hypertension. Kidney Int S59:S36–S38, 1997.

24. β-BLOCKERS

Ronald Flauto, D.O.

1. How do β-blockers reduce blood pressure (BP)?

An integrated explanation for the antihypertensive effect of β-blockers is lacking. Two major mechanisms seem most likely.

1. β-Blockers competitively inhibit the action of **catecholamines** on cardiac β-receptors with a consequent reduction in heart rate and cardiac output. The decrease in cardiac output occurs with acute and long-term β blockade and is associated with a decrease in arterial pressure.

2. β-Blockers suppress renin release from the juxtaglomerular cells. Suppression of the **renin-angiotensin-aldosterone system** probably accounts for their efficacy in hypertensive patients with increased plasma renin activity (PRA). β-Blockers decrease BP in patients with normal or suppressed PRA. This observation has led to speculation that additional mechanisms, such as resetting of the arterial baroreceptors or reduction of central sympathetic outflow, might explain their antihypertensive effect.

2. Discuss properties of β-blockers that are clinically important.

β-blockers with **intrinsic sympathomimetic activity** (ISA) exhibit partial agonist activity, which may be associated with a lower incidence of bradycardia. If a β-blocker is the appropriate antihypertensive agent, the task becomes choosing the best agent for the patient. Knowledge of the pharmacokinetics and pharmacodynamics is helpful. **Selectivity, lipophilicity,** and **clearance** are the clinically important attributes of these drugs.

β_1-receptors predominate in the heart, and β_2-receptors predominate in the bronchi. Stimulation of the β_1**-receptors** increases the heart rate and cardiac output, whereas stimulation of the β_2**-receptors** results in bronchodilation. Nonselective β-blockade can cause bradycardia, a decreased cardiac output, and bronchospasm. Increasing doses of even the β_1 selective agents result in less cardioselectivity. High doses of selective β-blockers can elicit some of the side effects seen with blockade of the β_2-receptors (e.g., bronchospasm).

Lipophilic β-blockers cross the blood-brain barrier. This characteristic allows the drug to restore vagal tone. The loss of vagal tone increases the risk of sudden death. Theoretically, cardioprotective efficacy may be associated with moderate-to-high lipophilicity. Clinical differences between lipophilic and hydrophilic β-blockers have not been shown in a comparative prospective, randomized trial. The ability to cross the blood-brain barrier can increase the known central nervous system side effects of these agents (see later).

The **dosing interval** has a clinical impact. Agents that can be used once daily increase adherence.

3. Summarize β-blockers used in BP reduction.

See table, next page.

GENERIC NAME (TRADE NAME)	β-1 SELECTIVITY	ISA	DOSING INTERVAL	DOSE RANGE (mg)
Acebutolol (Sectral)	X	X	Daily	200–800
Atenolol (Tenormin)	X		Daily	25–100
Betaxolol (Kerlone)	X		Daily	5–20
Bisoprolol (Zebeta)	X		Daily	2.5–10
Carteolol (Cartrol)		X	Daily	2.5–10
Carvedilol* (Coreg)			bid	†
Labetalol* (Normodyne)			bid	200–1200
Metoprolol (Lopressor)	X		bid‡	50–300
Nadolol (Corgard)			Daily	40–320
Penbutolol (Levatol)		X	Daily	10–20
Pindolol (Visken		X	bid	10–60
Propranolol (Inderal)			bid‡	40–480
Timolol (Blocadren)			bid	20–60

* α and β blocking activity.
† Dosing varies depending on disease process being treated.
‡ Long-acting, once-daily preparations are available.

4. How well do β-blockers reduce BP?

Decrease in BP is generally proportional to baseline BP. Data from five trials comparing β-blockers with thiazide diuretics showed a mean decrease in the BP of 24.3/15.2 mm Hg with β-blockers. This is slightly less than the reduction achieved with thiazide diuretics, the universally accepted first-line agents. Thiazide diuretics are more tolerable, however. In two trials comparing β-blockers with placebo, systolic BP was lowered a mean of 10.3 mm Hg and diastolic BP 5.7 mm Hg. Approximately 60% of treated essential hypertensives achieve goal BP with β-blockers as monotherapy, a rate similar to that seen with other classes of antihypertensive agents.

5. In which patients are β-blockers more effective?

Younger patients, whites, and patients with high PRA compared with older patients, blacks, and patients with low PRA.

6. Are β-blockers first-line agents for hypertension?

Yes. β-Blockers are recommended along with thiazide diuretics as first-line therapy for uncomplicated hypertension. β-blockers are recommended alone or in combination with a thiazide diuretic for the management of hypertension in patients < 60 years old. The comorbid conditions of the patients affect the selection.

7. Do β-blockers decrease cardiovascular morbidity and mortality?

It depends (see table, next page).

1. Prospective randomized trials show that β-blockers significantly decrease the risk of stroke and myocardial infarction in essential hypertensives < 65 years old. Cigarette smoking nullifies the beneficial effect of nonselective β blockade, however.

2. In hypertensive patients > 65 years old, β-blockers significantly decrease the risk of stroke but do not affect coronary heart disease morbidity or cardiovascular mortality appreciably. In the elderly, β-blockers are effective for **secondary** but not primary prevention of cardiovascular morbidity and mortality.

Prospective Trials Using Diuretics or Beta-blockers as First-line Therapy in Elderly Hypertensive Patients

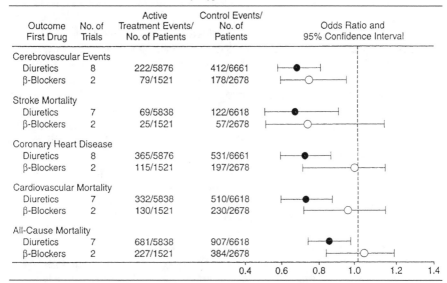

Outcome First Drug	No. of Trials	Active Treatment Events/ No. of Patients	Control Events/ No. of Patients	Odds Ratio and 95% Confidence Interval
Cerebrovascular Events				
Diuretics	8	222/5876	412/6661	
β-Blockers	2	79/1521	178/2678	
Stroke Mortality				
Diuretics	7	69/5838	122/6618	
β-Blockers	2	25/1521	57/2678	
Coronary Heart Disease				
Diuretics	8	365/5876	531/6661	
β-Blockers	2	115/1521	197/2678	
Cardiovascular Mortality				
Diuretics	7	332/5838	510/6618	
β-Blockers	2	130/1521	230/2678	
All-Cause Mortality				
Diuretics	7	681/5838	907/6618	
β-Blockers	2	227/1521	384/2678	

From Messerli FH, Grossman E, Goldbourt U: Are beta-blockers efficacious as first-line therapy for hypertension in the elderly? A systematic review. JAMA 279:1903–1907, 1991.

8. List the major clinical adverse reactions associated with β-blockers.

Fatigue	Hallucinations
Lethargy	Sinus bradycardia
Decreased exercise tolerance	Any degree of heart block
Sleep disturbance	Hypotension
Vivid dreams	Bronchospasm

9. How does tolerance of β-blockers compare with thiazide diuretics?

In one study, 10.3% of patients could not tolerate β-blockers because of side effects compared with 7.0% of patients receiving the diuretic. This was despite the exclusion of patients with asthma, sick sinus syndrome, sinus bradycardia, and atrioventricular block.

10. Discuss adverse metabolic effects of β-blockers.

Nonselective β-blockers without ISA decrease **high-density lipoprotein** (HDL) by 10% to 20% and increase **triglycerides** by 20% to 50%, whereas cardioselective β-blockers without ISA decrease HDL by 7% to 10% and increase triglycerides by 10% to 20%. Cardioselective β-blockers with ISA have the least effect on the lipid profile.

β-Blockade can increase **blood glucose**. Impaired glucose tolerance occurs more with nonselective compared with selective β-blockers. In diabetic patients, β-blockers can mask the hypoglycemic symptoms, so caution is advised when used in this setting.

Nonselective β-blockers can increase **serum potassium** by inhibition of β_2-mediated sodium-potassium transport in skeletal muscle. This effect is clinically insignificant except in patients who have other constraints on potassium homeostasis.

11. Are there any groups of patients in which β-blockers should be avoided?

β-Blockers are **contraindicated** in patients with second-degree or third-degree heart block. They should be avoided in patients with reactive airway disease or chronic obstructive lung disease, unless there are compelling indications.

The potential to mask hypoglycemic symptoms should prompt caution regarding the use of these agents in **diabetics**. Diabetics treated with β-blockers have a similar or greater reduction of total cardiovascular events and coronary heart disease, however, compared with nondiabetics, so the risks must be weighed against the benefits in this population.

In patients with **peripheral arterial occlusive disease**, it is possible to worsen symptoms caused by unopposed α constriction. This side effect is less with selective β-blockers and those with ISA.

β-Blockers are **pregnancy category C**.

12. How is labetalol different from other β-blockers?

Labetalol has selective, competitive α_1-adrenergic blocking properties as well as nonselective β-blocking properties. Hypotension, particularly orthostatic hypotension, is more common with this combination agent.

13. Name the advantages of labetalol.
  • Particularly useful in hypertensive urgencies because it can be administered in multiple intravenous aliquots over a relatively short period of time
  • Free of the side effects of nitroprusside
  • Can be used safely in renal failure

14. Discuss carvedilol.

Carvedilol is an α_1-adrenoreceptor blocker causing precapillary vasodilation and a nonselective β-blocker without ISA. The ratio of α-to-β blockade is about 1:10, whereas labetalol is roughly 1:4. There are fewer side effects compared with labetalol. Blood pressure control is similar to that obtained by labetalol, but carvedilol is not considered first-line therapy for hypertension because of cost. The primary use for carvedilol is congestive heart failure, particularly New York Heart Association class II or III.

15. List comorbid conditions that would favor selection of β-blockers compared with thiazide diuretics as first-line antihypertensive therapy.

Angina	Atrial fibrillation
Recent myocardial infarction	Recurrent migraine headache
Symptomatic systolic dysfunction	Hypertrophic obstructive cardiomyopathy

16. Is there any reason to use nonselective β-blockers in the treatment of hypertension?

Not really, unless cost is a major consideration. Selective β-blockers generally exhibit a better side-effect profile, and all are effective in a once-daily dosing regimen.

BIBLIOGRAPHY

1. Feldman RD, Campbell N, Larochelle P, et al: 1999 Canadian recommendations for the management of hypertension. Can Med Assoc J 161(suppl 12):S1–S17, 1999.
2. Fries ED: Current status of diuretics, beta-blockers, alpha-blockers and alpha-beta-blockers in the treatment of hypertension. Med Clin North Am 81:1305–1317, 1997.
3. Frishman WH: Carvedilol. N Engl J Med 339:1759–1765, 1998.
4. Joint National Committee on Prevention, Detection, Evaluation, and Treatment of High Blood Pressure: The Sixth Report of the Joint National Committee on Prevention, Detection, Evaluation, and Treatment of High Blood Pressure. Arch Intern Med 157:2413–2445, 1997.
5. Kendall MJ: Clinical relevance of pharmacokinetic differences between beta blockers. Am J Cardiol 80:15J–19J, 1997.
6. Messerli FH, Grossman E, Goldbourt U: Are beta-blockers efficacious as first-line therapy for hypertension in the elderly? A systematic review. JAMA 279:1903–1907, 1998.
7. SHEP Cooperative Research Group: Prevention of stroke by antihypertensive drug treatment in older persons with isolated systolic hypertension. JAMA 265:3255–3264, 1991.
8. Weir MR, Moser M: Diuretics and beta-blockers: Is there a risk for dyslipidemia? Am Heart J 139:173–184, 2000.
9. Wright JM: Choosing a first-line drug in the management of elevated BP: What is the evidence? 2. Beta-blockers. Can Med Assoc J 163:188–192, 2000.
10. Wright JM, Lee CH, Chambers GK: Systematic review of antihypertensive therapies: Does the evidence assist in choosing a first line drug? Can Med Assoc J 161:25–32, 1999.

25. α-BLOCKERS

Ronald Flauto, D.O.

1. How do α-adrenergic antagonists work?

There are two types of α-adrenoreceptors, α_1 and α_2. Presynaptic receptors are composed of the α_2 subtype, whereas postsynaptic receptors are α_1 and α_2 (see figure). Postsynaptic α_2-receptors are probably extrasynaptic and respond to circulating catecholamines rather than norepinephrine (NE) released from the sympathetic nerve. Stimulation of presynaptic α_2-receptors decreases NE release from postganglionic sympathetic nerve terminals. Binding of NE or epinephrine to vascular postsynaptic α_1-adrenoreceptors and α_2-adrenoreceptors results in vasoconstriction. Competitive binding of nonselective and selective α-adrenoreceptor blockers to postsynaptic receptors vasodilates resistance vessels in the peripheral circulation, decreases total peripheral resistance and reduces blood pressure (BP).

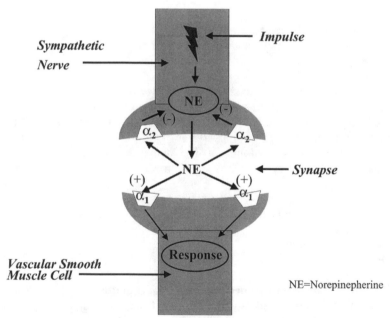

NE=Norepinepherine

2. What are some examples of α-blockers?

Some of the first available α-blockers, such as **phentolamine** and **phenoxybenzamine**, were **nonselective**. Their long-term use was limited by significant side effects, such as reflex tachycardia and salt and water retention. To limit the side effects, **selective α_1-adrenergic antagonists** were developed; these include **prazosin, doxazosin**, and **terazosin**. Only selective α_1-blockers currently are used for long-term treatment of hypertension.

3. Give guidelines for administration of α-blockers.

GENERIC NAME (TRADE NAME)	α_1 SELECTIVITY	DOSING INTERVAL	DOSE RANGE (mg)
Pentolamine* (Regitine)		Titrated to blood pressure	Bolus or infusion
Phenoxybenzamine[†] (Dibenzyline)		bid–tid	10.0–40.0
Prazosin (Minipress)	X	bid–tid	1.0–20.0
Terazosin (Hytrin)	X	qd–bid	1.0–20.0
Doxazosin (Cardura)	X	qd	1.0–16.0

* Perioperative management of pheochromocytoma.
[†] Preoperative management of pheochromocytoma.
bid = twice a day; tid = three times a day; qd = every day.

4. Are selective α-blockers considered first-line agents for hypertension?

No, because no data are available, in contrast to evidence for diuretics and β-blockers, to show that α-adrenoreceptor blockers decrease cardiovascular morbidity and mortality.

5. How well do α-blockers lower BP?

Prazosin, terazosin, and doxazosin reduce BP to a similar degree compared with β-blockers, thiazide diuretics, and angiotensin-converting enzyme inhibitors.

6. What is the most common side effect of selective α-blockers?

Orthostatic hypotension, an effect that most often occurs after the first dose. This side effect, noted in initial trials with prazosin, is probably consequent to venodilation. Initiating therapy with low doses of 0.5 to 1 mg of prazosin at bedtime minimizes the first-dose phenomenon. The incidence of this effect decreases with continued administration and is less common with the longer acting agents, terazosin and doxazosin.

7. List other frequently reported adverse reactions of selective α-blockers.
Dizziness
Reflex tachycardia
Headache

8. Discuss a-blockers with special properties or unique uses.

Labetalol is a combined α- and β-blocker. The β-blocking properties are nonselective, and its moderate α_1-receptor antagonism wanes with time. As a result, labetalol should be considered a β-blocker and is discussed in more detail in Chapter 24.

Phentolamine and **phenoxybenzamine** are indicated exclusively for treatment of hypertension in patients with **pheochromocytoma**. Phentolamine has a short half-life and is available only as a parenteral preparation. It is useful in BP control in the perioperative period. Phenoxybenzamine, an orally available nonselective α-blocker, can be used for preoperative management of hypertensive patients with pheochromocytoma. Use of phenoxybenzamine has decreased with the availability of α_2-agonists and calcium channel blockers.

9. What classes of antihypertensive agents can be combined with α-blockers?

Diuretics are effective in combination with α-blockers because α-blockers induce salt and water retention consequent to activation of the renin-angiotensin-aldosterone system. The antihypertensive effect is additive. The combination may counteract any deleterious effects on the lipid profile induced by thiazide diuretics.

β-Blockers are effective in combination with α-blockers because α-blockers may counteract any negative effect on the lipid profile or unopposed α-mediated constriction of the peripheral blood vessels induced by β blockade. β-Blockers can prevent reflex tachycardia resulting from α-adrenoreceptor antagonism.

10. Are there any specific contraindications to α-blockers?

No. The Antihypertensive and Lipid-Lowering Treatment to Prevent Heart Attack Trial (ALLHAT) results suggest a **restricted use** in hypertensive patients with **cardiovascular disease** (see Question 13). **Caution** should be used in the elderly who are prone to **orthostatic hypotension**.

11. List comorbid conditions that might benefit from α blockade.

Benign prostatic hypertrophy. α-Blockers are indicated for this condition in normotensive patients.

Dyslipidemia. Treatment with selective α_1-adrenoreceptor antagonists reduces total cholesterol, increases high-density lipoprotein (HDL) cholesterol, and decreases the total cholesterol-to-HDL ratio.

12. Summarize the use of α-blockers in hypertension.

1. They are not first-line agents in uncomplicated essential hypertension.

2. They can be used as first-line therapy to treat hypertension in patients with specific comorbidities:

    a. Hypercholesterolemia

    b. Prostatic hypertrophy

3. They should not be used as first-line agents in older high-risk hypertensive patients.

CONTROVERSY

13. Discuss the ALLHAT study and its preliminary findings.

ALLHAT randomized >40,000 hypertensive patients ≥55 years old with at least one additional coronary heart disease (CHD) risk factor to treatment with a diuretic (chlorthalidone), calcium channel antagonist (amlodipine), angiotensin-converting enzyme inhibitor (lisinopril), or α-adrenergic blocker (doxazosin) as initial antihypertensive therapy. Additional agents could be added to achieve a goal BP of <140/90 mm Hg. The primary end point was fatal CHD or nonfatal myocardial infarction (MI). Secondary end points included stroke and combined cardiovascular disease (CVD) composed of CHD death, nonfatal MI, angina, congestive heart failure (CHF), coronary revascularization, and peripheral vascular disease. Follow-up was planned for 4 to 8 years. After a median of 3.3 years, the doxazosin treatment arm was terminated on recommendation of the ALLHAT Data Safety Monitoring Board (DSMB).

An interim analysis by the DSMB showed that, compared with the chlorthalidone arm, the doxazosin group showed a higher risk of combined CVD (RR, 1.25; $P<.001$) and stroke (RR, 1.19; $P=.04$). The greater risk of combined CVD was driven primarily by a doubling of CHF in the doxazosin group (RR, 2.04; $P<.001$) but also was significant with regard to angina (RR, 1.16; $P<.001$) and coronary revascularization (RR, 1.15; $P=.05$). There were no differences between chlorthalidone and doxazosin with regard to the primary end points of fatal CHD or nonfatal MI. Throughout the study, mean systolic BP was 2 to 3 mm Hg higher in the doxazosin group, an observation that could account for the difference in stroke and angina but not the remarkable increase in CHF.

14. Do these findings mean that selective α-blockers increase a hypertensive patient's risk of CHF?

Not necessarily. There was no placebo arm in the ALLHAT study. It cannot be concluded that doxazosin increases CHF risk compared with placebo. The difference in CHF rates between the diuretic and α-blocker group could be due to a deleterious effect of α-blockade when used as initial antihypertensive therapy in these high-risk patients. Initial antihypertensive therapy with diuretics (also used to treat CHF) might ameliorate signs and symptoms of CHF in predisposed individuals and account for the discrepancy.

BIBLIOGRAPHY

1. ALLHAT officers and coordinators for the ALLHAT collaborative research group: Major cardiovascular events in hypertensive patients randomized to doxazosin vs. chlorthalidone. The Antihypertensive and Lipid-Lowering Treatment to Prevent Heart Attack Trial. JAMA 283:1967–1975, 2000.
2. Feldman RD, Campbell N, Larochelle P, et al: 1999 Canadian recommendations for the management of hypertension. Can Med Assoc J 161:S1–S17, 1999.
3. Fries ED: Current status of diuretics, beta-blockers, alpha-blockers, and the alpha-beta-blockers in the treatment of hypertension. Med Clin North Am 81:1305–1317, 1997.
4. Joint National Committee on Prevention, Detection, Evaluation, and Treatment of High Blood Pressure: The sixth report of the Joint National Committee on Prevention, Detection, Evaluation, and Treatment of High Blood Pressure. Arch Intern Med 157:2413–2445, 1997.
5. Kincaid-Smith PS: Alpha blockade: An overview of efficacy data. Am J Med 82:218–255, 1987.
6. van Zwieten PA: Alpha-adrenoreceptor blocking agents in the treatment of hypertension. In Laragh JH, Brenner BM (eds): Hypertension: Pathophysiology, Diagnosis, and Management. New York, Raven Press, 1995, pp 2917–2935.

26. CALCIUM CHANNEL BLOCKERS

Michael C. Smith, M.D.

1. How do calcium channel blockers (CCBs) lower blood pressure?

All currently available CCBs bind to the α_{1c} subunit of the L-type (voltage-gated) calcium channel and inhibit transmembrane calcium flux. The resulting decrease in cytosolic free calcium causes relaxation of vascular smooth muscle, vasodilation, a decrease in total peripheral resistance, and a consequent reduction in blood pressure.

2. Are there different classes of CCBs?

There are three classes of CCBs available for treatment of hypertension, the phenylalkylamines, benzothiazepines, and the dihydropyridines. Examples of available CCBs along with dosing guidelines are shown in the table.

CLASS	GENERIC NAME	DOSING INTERVAL*	DOSE RANGE (mg)†
Phenylalkylamine	Verapamil		
	Immediate Release	TID	120–480
	Sustained Release	QD–BID	120–480
Benzothiazepine	Diltiazem		
	Immediate Release	TID	60–360
	Sustained Release	QD	180–360
Dihydropyridine	Nifedipine	QD	30–120
	Amlodipine	QD	2.5–10
	Felodipine	QD	2.5–10
	Isradipine	BID	2.5–10
	Nicardipine	QD	60–120
	Nisoldipine	QD	20–40

* To encourage adherence, drugs that have a QD dosing regimen are recommended.
† Dosages should be individualized by titration of antihypertensive effect.

3. Do the various classes of CCBs differ in their cardiac effects?

Yes. Although a reduction in cytosolic calcium in cardiac muscle in vitro results in negative inotropic and chronotropic effects, this is apparent clinically only with the nondihydropyridine CCBs. The dihydropyridine CCBs, on the other hand, activate the sympathetic nervous system to varying degrees, thus attenuating their negative inotropic and chronotropic effects.

4. Are CCBs first-line therapy for the treatment of hypertension?

This is an unsettled issue. According to the Sixth Report of the Joint National Committee on Prevention, Detection, Evaluation, and Treatment of High Blood Pressure (JNC VI), only diuretics and β-blockers are recommended as first-line therapy for uncomplicated hypertension. Nevertheless, JNC VI recognizes that there may be specific or compelling indications for the use of CCBs. Under these circumstances, antihypertensive drugs are used not only to lower blood pressure but to favorably influence comorbid conditions. For CCBs, these indications are:

- Specific Indications
  Angina
  Atrial tachycardia and fibrillation (nondihydropyridine)
  Migraine (nondihydropyridine)
  Cyclosporine-induced hypertension
- Compelling Indications
  Isolated systolic hypertension (ISH) (long-acting dihydropyridines)

In the near future, data from studies such as the Antihypertensive and Lipid-Lowering Treatment to Prevent Heart Attack Trial (ALLHAT) comparing chlorthalidone, lisinopril, doxazosin, and amlodipine in the treatment of older, high-risk hypertensive patients will clarify the role of CCBs as first-line antihypertensive therapy.

5. Why are long-acting dihydropyridine CCBs indicated in the treatment of ISH?

First of all, diuretics are still preferred for patients with ISH. However, data from the Systolic Hypertension in Europe Trial (SYST-EUR) showed that an antihypertensive regimen based on nitrendipine, a dihydropyridine CCB unavailable in the United States, significantly decreased the risk of cerebrovascular morbidity and mortality compared with placebo. Further, ISH occurs predominantly in patients over the age of 60, a "low renin" hypertensive population in whom CCBs are particularly effective.

6. What factors predict a favorable antihypertensive response to CCBs?

- Older age
- Black race
- Low plasma renin activity (PRA)

Since blacks and the elderly demonstrate a high prevalence of low-renin hypertension, there is some redundancy to this classification. In addition, there is broad overlap

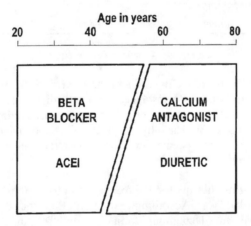

Schematic representation of monotherapy for patients with essential hypertension as a function of age and plasma renin activity (PRA). In general, ACE inhibitors and β-blockers are more effective in younger patients with high PRA, whereas diuretics and CCBs exhibit greater efficacy in older patients with low PRA. (From Buhler FK: Antihypertensive Care with Calcium Antagonists. In Laragh JH, Brenner BM [eds]: Hypertension: Pathophysiology, Diagnosis, and Management. New York, Raven Press, 1995, pp. 2801–2814, with permission.)

in the response of various demographic groups to different classes of antihypertensive agents. Nevertheless, both CCBs and diuretics demonstrate particular efficacy in hypertensive patients with low PRA.

7. What is the role of CCBs in the treatment of renal parenchymal hypertension?

The place of CCBs in treating hypertension in patients with declining renal function is a work in progress. These drugs have enjoyed widespread application in this patient population because some, but not all, studies demonstrated a greater renoprotective effect compared with other classes of antihypertensive agents. Further, since CCBs, in contrast to other classes of antihypertensive drugs, are effective at extremes of dietary salt intake (see figure), they are especially effective in salt-dependent hypertension.

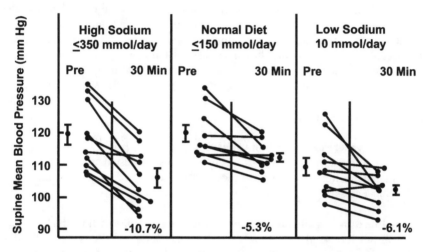

Change in mean supine blood pressure after administration of nifedipine in 10 patients with essential hypertension after 5 days of a high, normal or low sodium diet. (From MacGregor GA et al. Am J Nephrol 7:44–48, 1987, with permission.)

Recent data, however, have tempered enthusiasm for CCBs as first-line treatment in hypertensive patients with renal dysfunction. An interim analysis of the African American Study of Kidney Disease and Hypertension (AASK) found that ramipril was more effective than amlodipine in slowing the decline in renal function in blacks with hypertensive nephropathy and proteinuria > 300 mg/day. Consequently, the CCB arm of the trial was terminated. Moreover, a preliminary report recently showed that irbesartan was superior to both amlodipine and placebo in retarding the progression of renal disease in type II diabetic nephropathy.

Taken together, the data suggest a limited role for long-acting dihydropyridine CCBs as first-line therapy in hypertensive patients with renal dysfunction. On the other hand, nondihydropyridine CCBs lower proteinuria and may have an independent renoprotective effect. In the final analysis, CCBs should be reserved for third-line therapy (after diuretics and ACE inhibitors or angiotensin II receptor blockers) in the majority of hypertensive patients with renal disease.

8. Do CCBs decrease cardiovascular morbidity and mortality?

Recent meta-analyses have demonstrated that CCBs decrease the risk of stroke, major cardiovascular events, and cardiovascular death compared with placebos. In addition, they exhibit a similar effect on stroke and all cause mortality compared with diuretics, β-blockers, and ACE inhibitors. However, they do not reduce the risk of myocardial infarction, congestive heart failure, or major cardiovascular events compared with diuretics, β-blockers, or ACE inhibitors. In fact, one meta-analysis found that CCBs actually increased the risk of these events compared with the latter antihypertensive classes. Therefore, CCBs should be used cautiously in patients at increased risk of coronary artery disease and congestive heart failure.

9. Do CCBs increase the risk of myocardial infarction in hypertensive diabetics?

Probably not. This concern stems from the fact that several trials demonstrated that hypertensive diabetics treated with ACE inhibitors had a significantly lower risk of fatal and nonfatal myocardial infarction and cardiovascular events compared with those treated with long-acting dihydropyridine CCBs. However, this observation might be due to the fact that ACE inhibitors confer an additional protective effect with regard to cardiovascular events rather than the result of a deleterious effect of CCBs. Nevertheless, given the evidence to date, CCBs should not be the first-choice antihypertensive for diabetics.

10. Do CCBs increase the risk of cancer?

No. Although several early retrospective studies suggested an increased risk of cancer in patients treated with CCBs, recent studies concluded that CCBs are not related to cancer risk.

11. Are there any significant drug or dietary interactions with CCBs?

Yes. Both verapamil and diltiazem inhibit the clearance of drugs metabolized by the cytochrome P-450 CYP3A enzyme system. Hence, they should be used cautiously with drugs that undergo biotransformation by this system (e.g., carbamazepine, cyclosporine, HMG-CoA reductase inhibitors, HIV-protease inhibitors, etc.). In general, this same interaction is not found with the dihydropyridine CCBs. However, ingestion of large amounts of grapefruit juice can increase the bioavailability of the dihydropyridine CCBs.

12. What are some clinically important side effects of the CCBs?

As a class CCBs do not demonstrate any adverse biochemical effects. Common side effects associated with these drugs include edema, flushing, and headache (dihydropyridines); and constipation, bradycardia, or increasing heart block (diltiazem, verapamil).

13. Are short-acting CCBs indicated for the treatment of hypertension?

No. Initially, short-acting CCBs (e.g., nifedipine) were used for the long-term treatment of hypertension and employed sublingually to treat hypertensive urgencies; however, they can no longer be recommended. Short-acting CCBs cause excessive activation of the sympathetic nervous system and have been linked to excess cardiovascular morbidity and mortality.

14. What is the current role for CCBs in the treatment of hypertension?
- Not first-line therapy for uncomplicated essential hypertension
- Can be used as first line treatment for patients with specific or compelling indications:
    Supraventricular tachyarrhythmias
    Migraine
    Isolated systolic hypertension
- Use cautiously in patients at risk for coronary artery disease or congestive heart failure
- Excellent adjunctive agents for:
    Renal parenchymal hypertension
    Resistant hypertension

REFERENCES
1. Abernethy DR, Schwartz JB: Calcium-antagonist drugs. N Engl J Med 341:1447–1457, 1999.
2. Agodoa LY, Appel L, Bakris GL, et al: Effect of ramipril vs amlodipine on renal outcomes in hypertensive nephrosclerosis: A randomized controlled trial. J Am Med Assoc 285:2719–2728, 2001.
3. Alderman MH, Cohen H, Roque R, Madhavan S: Effect of long-acting and short-acting calcium antagonists on cardiovascular outcomes in hypertensive patients. Lancet 349:594–598, 1997.
4. Blood Pressure Lowering Treatment Trialists' Collaboration: Effects of ACE inhibitors, calcium antagonists, and other blood-pressure-lowering drugs: results of prospectively designed overviews of randomised trials. Lancet 356:1955–1964, 2000.
5. Buhler FK: Antihypertensive Care with Calcium Antagonists. In Laragh JH, Brenner BM (eds): Hypertension: Pathophysiology, Diagnosis and Management. New York, Raven Press, 1995, pp 2801–2814.
6. Cohen HJ, Pieper CF, Hanlon JT, et al: Calcium channel blockers and cancer. Am J Med 108:210–215, 2000.
7. Estacio RO, Jeffers BW, Hiatt WR, et al: The effect of nisoldipine as compared with enalapril on cardiovascular outcomes in patients with non-insulin dependent diabetes and hypertension. N Engl J Med 338:645–652, 1998.
8. He J, Whelton PK: Selection of initial antihypertensive drug therapy. Lancet 356:1942–1943, 2000.
9. Pahor M, Psaty BM, Alderman MH, et al: Health outcomes associated with calcium antagonists compared with other first-line antihypertensive therapies: A meta-analysis of randomised controlled trials. Lancet 356:1949–1954, 2000.

27. PERIPHERAL ADRENERGIC INHIBITORS, CENTRALLY ACTING SYMPATHOLYTICS, AND VASODILATORS

*Andrew S. O'Connor, D.O., Michael Patterson, D.O.,
and Michael C. Smith, M.D.*

1. What are the major anatomic structures in the efferent sympathetic nervous system? What neurotransmitters are involved in the transmission of impulses?

Central adrenergic efferent impulses pass through the major cardiovascular centers located in the hypothalamus, medulla (within the nucleus tractus solitarii), and subcortical areas within the spinal cord. They then synapse at the sympathetic chain ganglia located within the thoracolumbar area, where impulses are mediated by the release of acetylcholine. Peripherally, at the site of action of the postganglionic sympathetic fibers, neurotransmission is mediated by the release of norepinephrine, which binds to both α and β receptors, thus increasing both total peripheral resistance (TPR) and cardiac output (CO).

2. Aside from the direct action of vasoconstriction and increase in cardiac output, what other effects of chronic sympathetic hyperactivity contribute to hypertension?

Investigators have demonstrated that a rise in sympathetic activity parallels increased activity of the renin-angiotensin-aldosterone system (RAAS). Stimulation of the RAAS augments blood pressure by two additional mechanisms. First, angiotensin II is a potent vasoconstrictor and directly increases TPR. Second, both angiotensin II and aldosterone decrease salt and water excretion and contribute to volume-mediated increases in blood pressure.

3. Where along the neural pathway can the action of the sympathetic nervous system be blocked? What are examples of agents that work in each location?

Commonly Used Peripheral Adrenergic Inhibitors and Centrally Acting Sympatholytics

GENERIC NAME	TRADE NAME	DOSING INTERVAL	DOSE RANGE (mg)*
Peripheral adrenergic inhibitors			
Guanadrel	Hylorel	bid–tid	0–75
Guanethadine	Ismelin	qd	10–150
Reserpine[†]	Serpasil	qd	0.05–0.25
Centrally acting α_2 agonists			
Clonidine	Catapres	bid	0.2–1.2
Clonidine transdermal	Catapres-TTS	Weekly	0.1–0.3
Guanabenz	Wytensin	bid	8–32
Guanfacine	Tenex	qd	1–3
Methyldopa	Aldomet	bid	500–3000

* Dosages should be individualized by titration of antihypertensive effect.
[†] Also acts centrally.
bid = twice a day; tid = three times a day; qd = each day.

Peripheral adrenergic inhibitors. As a class, these agents act by binding to receptors on the postganglionic axon. They have no effect on the release of acetylcholine itself. However, because of their potent blockade of the sympathetic nervous system (SNS), they often are associated with unwanted and unopposed parasympathetic activity. These drugs decrease heart rate, reduce myocardial contractility, and lower peripheral vascular resistance. Further, because of the reduction in sympathetic tone, they decrease central venous return due to vasodilation of capacitance vessels. An example of this is reserpine, which both depletes the nerve terminal of norepinephrine and prevents the reuptake of norepinephrine. Unfortunately, this drug also depletes the central nervous system (CNS) of catecholamines and serotonin, a phenomenon that has been linked to psychomotor retardation and depression. As a result of inhibition of the SNS, reserpine is associated with relative parasympathetic hyperactivity manifested as bradycardia, atrioventricular node blockade, and occasionally extreme nasal stuffiness.

Preganglionic blocking agents. These medications exert their antihypertensive effect through stimulation of α_2 receptors within the major pathways of central sympathetic outflow or by blockade of the action of norepinephrine at its site of action. Examples of these medications include methyldopa and clonidine. Methyldopa is structurally related to dopa, the precursor of norepinephrine. Because of the structural homology, it is incorporated into the synthetic pathway and serves as a false neurotransmitter. More importantly, both methyldopa and clonidine stimulate α_2 receptors within the CNS, resulting in decreased central sympathetic tone, reduced brain turnover of norepinephrine, diminished central sympathetic outflow, and a consequent reduction in blood pressure.

4. Name the specific clinical situations in which the use of centrally acting antihypertensives is efficacious.

In the presence of **left ventricular hypertrophy** (LVH). Multiple studies have shown that LVH is an independent risk factor for cardiovascular morbidity and mortality. Although several classes of antihypertensive agents lower blood pressure as effectively as the centrally acting agents, this class of medications might induce regression of LVH through mechanisms independent of a reduction in blood pressure. This is probably the consequence of decreased sympathetic tone because increased activity of the SNS augments ventricular mass independent of an increase in blood pressure. Regression of LVH induced by centrally acting sympatholytics enhances LV diastolic function.

In the treatment of **renovascular and renal parenchymal hypertension**. Overactivity of the SNS occurs both in the presence of renal artery stenosis and in chronic renal insufficiency. Although the hypertension associated with both of these conditions is likely multifactorial, two studies demonstrated that, in patients with renal parenchymal hypertension, sympathetic postganglionic nerve discharge is significantly increased compared with controls. In addition, recent data have clearly shown that afferent sympathetic nerve traffic from diseased kidneys signals the CNS with a consequent increase in peripheral sympathetic nerve activity. Hence, these drugs are particularly useful in this difficult-to-treat patient population. Centrally acting antihypertensive agents also demonstrate a relatively "renal neutral" profile in terms of their effects on glomerular filtration rate and renal plasma flow.

In the treatment of **hypertension in diabetic patients**. As a class, these agents have a neutral to somewhat favorable effect on lipid profiles. They also have little effect on fasting glucose levels or hemoglobin A_{1C} levels.

5. What are the major side effects of the centrally acting antihypertensives?

Due to blockade of CNS sympathetic outflow, this class of medications causes a number of side effects that limit their utility as monotherapy in the treatment of hypertension. Their therapeutic range is narrow, and limiting side effects such as fatigue, dry mouth, and sexual dysfunction are frequent. Other important side effects include the potential to cause varying degrees of AV nodal block, an effect that is often additive when beta-blocking agents are used concomitantly.

An important and potentially life-threatening effect is the **discontinuation syndrome**, which occurs when large doses of these medications are stopped abruptly rather than tapered gradually. This syndrome is consequent to rebound overactivity of the SNS and is characterized by anxiety, tachycardia, and hypertension with blood pressures occasionally exceeding pretreatment levels.

6. What is antihypertensive escape and how does this relate to the use of centrally acting antihypertensive agents as monotherapy in the treatment of hypertension?

When these medications are used as monotherapy, they cause salt and water retention resulting in expansion of the extracellular fluid volume and a consequent attenuation of antihypertensive efficacy. This phenomenon is known as **pseudotolerance**. Therefore, these drugs generally need to be used in combination with a thiazide diuretic or low-dose loop-blocking agent to avoid this phenomenon and maintain smooth blood pressure control.

7. Are any of these drugs first-line antihypertensive agents?

Definitely not. Because of their significant side-effect profile and tendency to cause pseudotolerance, both peripheral adrenergic inhibitors and centrally acting sympatholytics are considered third- or fourth-line adjuncts in resistant hypertension or under special circumstances (e.g., renal insufficiency).

8. What antihypertensive agents are considered direct vasodilators?

Virtually all available antihypertensive agents reduce blood pressure by dilating resistance vessels thereby decreasing TPR and can be strictly considered vasodilators. For most, however, the mechanism of action involves decreasing the concentration of a known vasoconstrictor (e.g., angiotensin-converting enzyme inhibitor), blocking receptors for constrictor agonists (e.g., angiotensin II receptor blockers, α_1 blockers), or inhibiting calcium transients across cell membranes (e.g., calcium channel blockers). Consequently, these agents are not considered direct vasodilators. Direct vasodilators include nitroglycerin, sodium nitroprusside, diazoxide, hydralazine and minoxidil (see table, top of next page).

9. How do direct vasodilators reduce blood pressure?

The nitrovasodilators (nitroglycerin and sodium nitroprusside) increase the concentration of nitric oxide (NO), augment intracellular cyclic guanosine monophosphate

GENERIC NAME	TRADE NAME	DOSING INTERVAL	DOSE RANGE*
Nitroglycerin[†]		IV infusion	5–100 µg/min
Sodium nitroprusside[†]	Nipride	IV infusion	0.3–10 µg/kg/min
Diazoxide[†]	Hyperstat	IV infusion or IV bolus	15–30 mg/min/infusion 50–100 mg/bolus
Hydralazine	Apresoline	bid	50–300 mg/day
Minoxidil	Loniten	bid	5–100 mg/day

* Dosages should be individualized by titration of antihypertensive effect.
[†] Parenteral use only.
bid = twice a day.

(cGMP), and, hence, relax vascular smooth muscle with a resultant decrease in TPR. On the other hand, despite extensive investigation, the mode of action of diazoxide, hydralazine, and minoxidil remains poorly understood. Minoxidil might exert its vasodilator effect, in part, by opening potassium channels.

10. Which agents can be used for long-term treatment of hypertension?

Nitrovasodilators and diazoxide are used parenterally for hypertensive crises and, thus, are not indicated for chronic antihypertensive therapy (see Chapter 22). However, the advent of the nitrovasodilators has reduced the popularity of diazoxide, and it is currently used rarely, if at all. On the other hand, hydralazine and minoxidil are still employed as long-term antihypertensive agents.

11. Are hydralazine and minoxidil first-line agents for the treatment of hypertension?

No. Both hydralazine and minoxidil increase activity of the SNS and stimulate the RAAS. The net result is a reflex increase in heart rate and cardiac output and avid renal salt and water retention. These neurohumoral responses limit their use as monotherapy and require the addition of a sympatholytic agent and diuretic as part of the antihypertensive regimen.

12. When are hydralazine and minoxidil indicated in the treatment of hypertension?

Good question. Given the plethora of equally effective drugs with a superior side-effect profile, these agents are now used as fourth-line agents in patients intolerant of other drug classes or in those with the most resistant form of hypertension.

13. What are the major side effects of hydralazine?

The most common adverse reactions to hydralazine are a direct extension of its direct vasodilation and include headache, tachycardia, flushing, and dizziness. Less common side effects consist of gastrointestinal intolerance, hemolytic anemia, and a reversible syndrome of lupus erythematosus. The syndrome of drug-induced lupus usually occurs after prolonged therapy with doses above 200 mg per day in patients with the slow acetylator phenotype.

14. What side effects are usually seen with minoxidil?

Hypertrichosis is the most common side effect. Although this adverse effect generally makes the drug intolerable to women and children, it has been put to therapeutic advantage in a topical preparation to treat alopecia. Other side effects, like those of hydralazine, are a direct extension of its potent vasodilating effects with consequent stimulation of the SNS and RAAS and include tachycardia, headache, angina, and flushing. Also, the development of pericardial effusion has been well-described. The etiology is uncertain but may be the result of avid renal salt and water retention.

BIBLIOGRAPHY

1. Alpert MA, Bauer JH: Rapid control of severe hypertension with minoxidil. Arch Intern Med 142:2099–2104, 1982.
2. Converse R, Jacobsen TN, Toto RD, et al: Sympathetic overactivity in patients with chronic renal failure. N Engl J Med 327:1917–1921, 1992.
3. Lees KR, Reed JL: The pharmacology of antihypertensive erugs and drug-drug interactions. In Laragh JH, Brenner BM (eds): Hypertension: Pathophysiology, Diagnosis, and Management, 2nd ed. New York, Raven Press, 1995, pp 2985–2995.
4. Ligtenberg G, Blankestijn PJ, Oey PL, et al: Reduction of sympathetic hyperactivity by enalapril in patients with chronic renal failure. N Engl J Med 340:1321–1328, 1999.
5. Linas SL, Nies AS: Minoxidil. Ann Intern Med 94:61–65, 1981.
6. Oster J, Epstein M: Use of centrally acting sympatholytic agents in the management of hypertension. Arch Intern Med 151:1638–1644, 1991.
7. Remuzzi G: Sympathetic overactivity in hypertensive patients with chronic renal disease. N Engl J Med 340:1360–1361, 1999.
8. Robinson BF, Benjamin N: Vasodilators. In Laragh JH, Brenner BM (eds): Hypertension: Pathophysiology, Diagnosis, and Management. New York, Raven Press, 1990, pp 2263–2274.
9. Weber M, Graettinger W, Cheung D: Centrally acting sympathetic inhibitors. In Laragh JH, Brenner BM (eds): Hypertension: Pathophysiology, Diagnosis, and Management. New York, Raven Press, 1990, pp 2251–2261.

28. ANGIOTENSIN-CONVERTING ENZYME INHIBITORS AND ANGIOTENSIN II RECEPTOR BLOCKERS

Janice G. Douglas, M.D., and Kaine C. Onwuzulike

1. Describe the renin-angiotensin system (RAS).

The RAS plays an integral role in both short-term and long-term blood pressure regulation. This system is activated by situations decreasing absolute or effective blood volume such as a sodium restriction, diuretic use, blood loss, congestive heart failure, and cirrhosis. It is equally responsive to circumstances that lower total peripheral resistance, such as vasodilators. The dominant effector of this pathway is angiotensin II (AII), formed by the cleavage of angiotensin I (AT$_1$) by angiotensin-converting enzyme (ACE). The critical role of AII in essential hypertension stems from its potent vasoconstrictor properties, effect on neurotransmission and volume regulation, and mitogenic properties.

2. What is the role of the RAS in the regulation of arterial blood pressure?

The RAS has long been recognized as an essential determinant of arterial blood pressure regulation. A decrease in effective circulating volume triggers activation of the RAS, which restores balance under normal circumstances. The chief effects of this system are mediated by AII through the AT$_1$ receptor. The major actions that influence blood pressure directly are illustrated in the figure. However, in the presence of excessive levels of AII, extreme elevations in blood pressure can result.

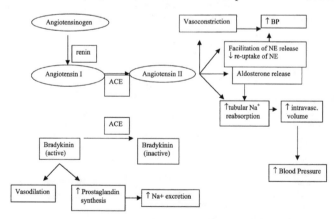

Schematic representation of the renin-angiotensin system and its role in blood pressure regulation.

3. Does angiotensin II have deleterious effects on cardiovascular and renal function independent of blood pressure?

Yes. In addition to its direct and indirect effects to increase blood pressure through both volume and vasoconstrictor-mediated mechanisms, AII is mitogenic, stimulates cardiovascular and renal remodeling, and is prothrombotic.

Angiotensin II Effects

PRESSOR EFFECTS	GROWTH PROMOTING EFFECTS	CARDIOVASCULAR AND RENAL REMODELING	MISCELLANEOUS
↑ Endothelin	Vascular smooth muscle proliferation	↑ Expression of protooncogenes	Superoxide production
↑ Vasopressin	Myocyte growth	↑ Synthesis of collegen and ECM proteins	Platelet aggregation
	Mesangial cell proliferation	↑ Production of TBF-β and other growth factors	↑ PAI 1/ thrombosis

4. What are the chemical structures and properties of ACE inhibitors?

ACE inhibitors first became available for the pharmacologic management of essential hypertension in the early 1980s. To date, nine compounds are approved in the U.S. for pharmacologic use (see table). ACE inhibitors are structurally heterogeneous and can be classified into three main categories based on differences in chemical structure:

1. Sulfhydryl-containing ACE inhibitors (e.g., captopril)
2. Dicarboxyl-containing ACE inhibitors (e.g., enalapril, lisinopril, benazapril)
3. Phosphorus-containing ACE inhibitors (e.g., fosinopril)

With the notable exception of fosinopril which is dually eliminated by the liver and kidney, ACE inhibitors are cleared predominantly by the kidneys. ACE inhibitors, with the exception of captopril and lisinopril, are prodrugs that require prior activation by the liver.

DRUG NAME	SULFHYDRYL GROUP	PHOSPHORUS GROUP	DICARBOXYL GROUP	RENAL ELIMINATION	PRODRUG
Moexipril			X	X	X
Benazepril			X	X	X
Captopril†‡	X			X	
Enalapril			X	X	X
Fosinopril*		X			X
Lisinopril†			X	X	
Quinapril			X	X	X
Ramipril			X	X	X
Perindopril				X	X

* Displays balanced elimination by liver and kidney.
† Active molecules that do not require activation.
‡ Directly stimulates prostaglandin synthesis.

5. How do ACE inhibitors lower blood pressure?

ACE inhibitors act in a dual fashion; they prevent the conversion of AT I, an inactive octapeptide, to AII and inhibit the degradation of bradykinin (see figure in question 2). Administration of ACE inhibitors does not significantly influence prostaglandin or catecholamine levels but does attenuate sympathetically mediated vasoconstriction without altering circulatory reflexes. This latter property explains why ACE inhibitors are rarely associated with postural hypotension unless the patient has a diminished plasma volume. In addition to causing systemic arteriolar dilatation, ACE inhibitors effectively increase arterial compliance, helping to lower blood pressure while maintaining cardiac output.

6. What are the currently available ACE inhibitors and recommended doses?

Recommended Dosages of Currently Available ACE Inhibitors

GENERIC NAME	TRADE NAME	DOSING INTERVAL	DOSE RANGE (MG)
Benazepril	Lotensin	qd–bid	5–40
Captopril	Capoten	bid–tid	12.5–150
Enalapril	Vasotec	qd–bid	2.5–40
Fosinopril	Monopril	qd	5–40
Lisinopril	Zestril/Prinivil	qd	5–40
Moexipril	Univasc	qd	7.5–15
Perindopril	Aceon	qd–bid	4–16
Quinapril	Accupril	qd–bid	10–80
Ramipril	Altace	qd–bid	1.25–20

qd = each day; bid = two times a day; tid = three times a day.

7. Describe the dose-response curve for ACE inhibitors.

The dose-response curve for ACE inhibitors with regard to reduction of blood pressure is fairly flat. The magnitude of the initial antihypertensive response tends to correlate directly with plasma renin activity (PRA) and plasma concentration of AII.

8. Describe the hemodynamic effects of ACE inhibitors.

Significant Hemodynamic Effects of ACE Inhibitors

HEMODYNAMIC PARAMETER	EFFECT
Mean arterial pressure	$\downarrow$
Peripheral vascular resistance	$\downarrow$
Cardiac output	$\uparrow \leftrightarrow$
Diastolic function	Usually improved
Renal plasma flow	$\uparrow$
Glomerular filtration rate[†]	$\leftrightarrow \downarrow$*
Efferent arteriolar compliance	$\uparrow$

* Due to preferential constriction of efferent glomerular arterioles > afferent arterioles by AII, administration of ACE inhibitors can cause an initial decrease in glomerular filtration rate.
[†] Contributes in part to renoprotective effects

9. What beneficial effects of ACE inhibitors extend beyond control of blood pressure?

In 1993, a landmark clinical trial documented the renoprotective effect (involving the composite clinical outcomes of dialysis or death) of captopril in insulin-dependent diabetics with overt nephropathy, an effect that was largely independent of reduction in blood pressure. Multiple lines of evidence from studies with less rigorous endpoints (surrogate outcomes such as decrease in proteinuria and slowing the decline in renal function) employing additional ACE inhibitors in patients with diabetic and nondiabetic renal disease also suggested important renoprotective effects that were independent of blood pressure. In addition, many large-scale clinical trials have documented that ACE inhibitors decrease morbidity and mortality in the setting of systolic dysfunction and post myocardial infarction. Cardioprotection has also been documented in high-risk patients treated with ramipril, an effect that was accompanied by a reduction in new-onset of diabetes.

10. Describe the common adverse effects of ACE inhibitors.

Adverse metabolic side effects are generally not encountered with administration of ACE inhibitors. In fact, some evidence exists that ACE inhibitors improve insulin sensitivity in patients with insulin resistance and decrease cholesterol and apolipoprotein A levels.

Major Adverse Effects of ACE Inhibitors

SIDE EFFECT	COMMENT
Hypotension	First dose phenomenon (usually in patients with renin-dependent hypertension)
Functional renal insufficiency	Initially described in bilateral renal artery stenosis or stenosis in a solitary kidney. However, 80-90% of all cases of ACE-induced acute renal failure occur in patients with chronic renal insufficiency, congestive heart failure (CHF), or volume depletion.
Hyperkalemia	Usually seen when used in combination with potassium-sparing diuretics or potassium supplements or in patients with other constraints on potassium homeostasis (i.e. renal insufficiency, diabetes, etc.).
Cough (5–20%)	Due to ($\uparrow$ bradykinin or substance P; women > men
Rash	Idiosyncratic reaction
Fetopathy	When administered past first trimester (AII via AT_2 receptors is required for normal fetal development)
Dysgeusia	May be attributable to sulfhydryl group on captopril and related ACE inhibitors (reversible upon discontinuation of ACE inhibitor).
Angioedema	Rare, sometimes fatal reaction usually occurring early in the course of ACE inhibition
Neutropenia	Rare but tends to occur in patients with collagen-vascular or renal parenchymal disease

11. Are there relevant drug interactions with ACE inhibitors?

- **Nonsteroidal anti-inflammatory drugs** (NSAIDs) can blunt the antihypertensive response to ACE inhibitors.
- **Potassium-sparing diuretics** or **potassium supplements** can cause hyperkalemia when used in conjunction with ACE inhibitors.
- ACE inhibitors increase plasma levels of **digoxin** and **lithium**.

12. Describe the synergistic relationship between ACE inhibitors and diuretics in the pharmacologic management of hypertension.

The antihypertensive effect of ACE inhibitors is most notably augmented with coadministration of a diuretic. Diuretics, via natriuresis, shift the hypertensive axis to a "renin-dependent" state, thereby increasing the efficacy of ACE inhibitors in the management of hypertension.

13. Describe the therapeutic utility of ACE inhibitors with β-blockers, sympatholytics and calcium channel blockers in the management of essential hypertension.

Combining β-blockers with an ACE inhibitor presumably blunts the hyperreninemia induced by ACE inhibitor therapy. However, this effect has been marginal thus far in clinical practice. On the other hand, ACE inhibitors demonstrate an additive response in lowering blood pressure when combined with an α-antagonist or calcium channel blocker.

14. Describe the mechanism of "ACE escape" with administration of an ACE inhibitor.

Although ACE inhibitors block the production of AII from angiotensin I, they do not curb the synthesis of AII by alternative pathways (e.g., chymase, cathepsin-sensitive angiotensin generating enzyme). Moreover, studies have documented that AII levels gradually return to baseline or higher after weeks to months of treatment with an ACE inhibitor. For this reason, angiotensin II receptor blockers (ARBs) provide more complete blockade of the RAS because the AT_1 receptor is blocked without the potential for bypassing access to this receptor.

15. What are the properties of ARBs?

ARBs, available in the United States since 1995, are nonpeptide imidazole-5-acetic acid derivatives with AT_1 receptor biospecificity. The first ARB developed was losartan. Similar to ACE inhibitors, the dose-response curve for ARBs is relatively shallow and correlates best with increments in the PRA.

16. What are the functions of the AT_1 and AT_2 receptor?

Major Functions of the AT_1 and AT_2 Receptors

AT_1	AT_2
Constantly expressed	Expressed primarily during fetal life and reexpressed during wound healing
Mediates vasoconstriction	Mediates vasodilation
Mediates trophic effects of AII (see above)	Mediates antimitogenic effects Nitric oxide activation

17. What are the mechanisms of action of ARBs?

All of the currently known actions of AII that influence blood pressure regulation are mediated by AII binding to the AT_1 receptor. The AT_2 receptor is expressed markedly during gestation. In the adult, AT_2 receptors have been best characterized in the kidney where they stimulate bradykinin and nitric oxide (NO) and have the potential to facilitate sodium excretion. Because the AT_1 receptor mediates inhibition of renin release, plasma renin activity (PRA) rises significantly during treatment with ARBs. Therefore, AII is free to bind to AT_2 receptors and potentially mediate vasodilation, exert antimitogenic effects, and stimulate NO synthesis. However, the extent to which AT_2 receptors contribute to beneficial effects of ARBs has as yet to be determined.

18. What are the currently available ARBs and recommended doses?

Currently Marketed ARBs and Dosing Recommendations

GENERIC NAME	TRADE NAME	DAILY DOSAGE (mg)
Candesartan	Atacand	8–32
Eprosartan	Teveten	400–800
Irbesartan	Avapro/Avalide*	150–300
Losartan	Cozaar/Hyzaar*	50–100
Telmisartan	Micardis*	20–80
Valsartan	Diovan/Diovan HCT*	80–320

* Available with hydrochlorothiazide.

19. What are the side effects of ARBs?

The virtual absence of symptomatic and metabolic side effects is an attractive feature of ARBs and provides a strong rationale for their use in patients who cannot tolerate ACE inhibitors or have type 2 diabetic nephropathy. Cough is not present with ARBs. However, hypotension and functional renal insufficiency occur to a similar extent as with ACE inhibitors. Hyperkalemia is less common compared with ACE inhibition. There have been rare reported cases of angioedema, and, like ACE inhibitors, ARBs should not be used during pregnancy. Similar to ACE inhibitors, the efficacy of ARBs is increased with prior administration of a diuretic.

20. What beneficial properties exist for ARBs compared with ACE inhibitors?

Unlike with ACE inhibitors, serum bradykinin and substance P levels are not affected by ARB administration, thereby eliminating the common side effect of dry cough seen with ACE inhibition.

An additional beneficial action unique to losartan is its uricosuric effect with a consequent reduction in serum uric acid. This property can be of therapeutic advantage in hypertensive patients with hyperuricemia.

Both ACE inhibitors and ARBs have the potential to produce hyperkalemia in patients with renal insufficiency because of inhibition of aldosterone production. However, ARBs have been documented to cause less hyperkalemia.

Several recent clinical trials have validated the beneficial effect of ARBs for renoprotection in type 2 diabetic nephropathy. Comparisons were between losartan and conventional therapy (RENAAL) and between irbesartan, amlodipine, and placebo (IDNT). In both studies, blood pressure was comparably controlled, but the ARBs were more renoprotective and demonstrated a significant decrease in composite clinical outcomes (end-stage renal disease, death, or doubling of serum creatinine).

21. Are ACE inhibitors or ARBs first-line antihypertensive therapy?

Not yet, but they may be soon. According to the Sixth Report of the Joint National Committee on Prevention, Detection, Evaluation, and Treatment of High Blood Pressure (JNC VI), diuretics and β-blockers are the drugs of choice for uncomplicated hypertension. Currently, ACE inhibitors and ARBs are recommended for patients with comorbid conditions that provide specific or compelling indications for their use. However, given the emerging data regarding both the cardioprotective and renoprotective effects of these two drug classes as well as the anticipated results of the Antihypertensive and Lipid-Lowering Treatment to Prevent Heart Attack Trial, we predict that one or both classes will be considered first-line treatment for essential hypertension in the near future.

BIBLIOGRAPHY

1. Bakris GL, Siomos M, Richardson D, et al, for the VAL-K Study Group: ACE inhibition or angiotensin receptor blockade: Impact on potassium in renal failure. Kidney Int 58:2084–2092, 2000.
2. Bauer JH, Reams GP: The angiotensin II type 1 receptor antagonists: A new class of antihypertensive drugs. Arch Intern Med 155:1361–1368, 1995.
3. The GISEN Group: Randomized, placebo-controlled trial of effect of ramipril on decline in glomerular filtration rate and risk of terminal renal failure in proteinuric nondiabetic nephropathy. Lancet 349:1857–1863, 1997.
4. Goodfriend TL, Elliott ME, Catt KJ: Angiotensin receptors and their antagonists. N Engl J Med 334:1649–1654, 1996.
5. Heart Outcomes Prevention Evaluation Study Investigators: Effects of an angiotensin-converting enzyme inhibitor, ramipril, on cardiovascular events in high-risk patients. N Engl J Med 342:145–153, 2000.
6. Hricik DE, Browning PJ, Kopelman R, et al: Captopril-induced functional renal insufficiency in patients with bilateral renal-artery stenoses or renal-artery stenosis in a solitary kidney. N Engl J Med 308:373–376, 1983.
7. Israili ZH, Hall WD: Cough and angioneurotic edema associated with angiotensin-converting enzyme inhibitor therapy. Ann Intern Med 117:234–242, 1992.
8. Lewis EJ, Hunsicker LG, Bain RP, Rohde RD, for the Collaborative Study Group: The effect of angiotensin-converting enzyme inhibition on diabetic nephropathy. N Engl J Med 329:1456–1462, 1993.
9. Shotan A, Widerhorn J, Hurst A, Elkayam U: Risks of angiotensin-converting enzyme inhibition during pregnancy: Experimental and clinical evidence, potential mechanisms, and recommendations for use. Am J Med 96:451–456, 1994.
10. Toto RD, Mitchell HC, Lee H-C, et al: Reversible renal insufficiency due to angiotensin converting enzyme inhibitors in hypertensive nephrosclerosis. Ann Intern Med 115:513–519, 1991.

29. APPLICATION OF THERAPEUTIC PRINCIPLES

Eleni Pelecanos, M.D., M.P.H.

1. What are components of cardiovascular risk stratification in patients with hypertension?

MAJOR RISK FACTORS	
Smoking	Sex (men and postmenopausal women)
Dyslipidemia	Family history of cardiovascular disease:
Diabetes mellitus	women < 65 or men < 55
Age > 60	

TARGET ORGAN DAMAGE/CLINICAL CARDIOVASCULAR DISEASE	
Heart diseases	Stroke or transient ischemic attack
Left ventricular hypertrophy	Nephropathy
Angina or prior myocardial infarction	Peripheral arterial disease
Prior coronary revascularization	Retinopathy
Heart failure	

From Joint National Committee on Prevention, Detection, Evaluation, and Treatment of High Blood Pressure: The Sixth Report of the Joint National Committee on Prevention, Detection, Evaluation, and Treatment of High Blood Pressure. Arch Intern Med 157:2413–2445, 1997.

2. List target systolic and diastolic BP for patients with coexisting conditions.

COMORBID CONDITION	BLOOD PRESSURE (mm Hg)
Diabetes	< 130/80
Renal failure without significant proteinuria	< 130/85
Renal failure with > 1 g proteinuria	< 125/75
No comorbid condition	< 140/90

3. When is a trial of lifestyle modification recommended in hypertensive patients?

If the patient is not at high risk and does not have systolic blood pressure (BP) > 159 mm Hg or diastolic BP > 99 mm Hg, a trial of lifestyle modification (e.g., low-salt diet, exercise) for several months is recommended before starting medication.

4. When should medication be prescribed in addition to recommending lifestyle modification to lower BP?

Consider the following factors:

1. The severity of the patient's hypertension relative to their goal BP
2. The presence of other cardiovascular risk factors
3. The presence and severity of target organ damage

The greater the combination of any of the above-listed factors, the greater the patient's risk of cardiovascular events, and the threshold to initiate treatment with medication should be lower.

5. Summarize risk stratification and treatment for hypertension.

BLOOD PRESSURE STAGES (mm Hg)	RISK GROUP A (No Risk Factors: No TOD/CCD)	RISK GROUP B (At Least 1 Risk Factor, Not Including Diabetes; No TOD/CCD)	RISK GROUP C (TOD/CCD and/or Diabetes, With or Without Other Risk Factors)
High–normal (130–139/85–89)	Lifestyle modification	Lifestyle modification	Drug therapy[†]
Stage 1 (140–159/90–99)	Lifestyle modification (up to 12 mo)	Lifestyle modification* (up to 6 mo)	Drug therapy
Stages 2 and 3 (≥ 160/≥ 100)	Drug therapy	Drug therapy	Drug therapy

NOTE: A patient with diabetes and a blood pressure of 142/94 mm Hg plus left ventricular hypertrophy should be classified as having stage 1 hypertension with target organ disease (left ventricular hypertrophy) and with another major risk factor (diabetes). This patient would be categorized as stage 1, risk group C and recommended for immediate initiation of pharmacologic treatment. Lifestyle modification should be adjunctive therapy for all patients recommended for pharmacologic therapy.
* For patients with multiple risk factors, clinicians should consider drugs as initial therapy plus lifestyle modifications
[†] For patients with heart failure, renal insufficiency, or diabetes.
TOD/CCD = Target organ disease/clinical cardiovascular disease.
From Joint National Committee on Prevention, Detection, Evaluation, and Treatment of High Blood Pressure: The Sixth Report of the Joint National Committee on Prevention, Detection, Evaluation, and Treatment of High Blood Pressure. Arch Intern Med 157:2413–2445, 1997.

6. What are the basic considerations in choosing a medication for a particular patient?

1. What is the evidence that the medication reduces cardiovascular and overall morbidity and mortality?

2. How likely is the medication to reduce the patient's BP effectively?

3. Is the medication well tolerated, easy to take, compatible with the patient's other conditions and medications, and accessible?

7. What patient demographics may help predict response to particular antihypertensives?

Remember the mnemonic BODE:
B Black
O Overweight
D Diabetic
E Elderly

8. Discuss the effectiveness of specific drugs in reducing BP in particular patients.

In general, the more **BODE** characteristics the patient has, the more likely they are to have more **salt-sensitive** hypertension, and they may be more likely to respond to **diuretics** or **calcium channel blockers** as initial therapy than to β-blockers or ACE inhibitors. Patients with fewer of these characteristics often have more **renin-driven** or **catecholamine-driven** hypertension and respond better to **ACE inhibitors** or **β-blockers** as monotherapy.

For **older** patients with isolated systolic hypertension, **diuretics** are the preferred agents (see Chapter 20).

In patients with **renal insufficiency** and creatinine clearances < 30 mL/min, thiazide diuretics often are ineffective. **Loop-blocking diuretics**, such as furosemide (given in a twice-a-day dosing regimen), generally are required to achieve optimal BP control, especially if the patient has evidence of volume overload (e.g., lower extremity edema).

9. Discuss other considerations in choosing antihypertensive medication.

Whether a medication is well tolerated, easy to take, compatible with the patient's other conditions and medications, and accessible is crucial to a patient's ability and willingness to adhere to the prescribed treatment.

Side effects should be minimal.

Medications that need to be taken **more than once a day** (especially for an asymptomatic condition such as hypertension) generally lead to poor compliance.

Consider the patient's **comorbid conditions** (e.g., diabetes, asthma, coronary artery disease, prostatic hypertrophy) and choose agents that may ameliorate or at least do not aggravate these conditions.

Consider the **availability** and **affordability** of the medication: If the patient can't get it, why bother prescribing it?

10. What are some common coindications for particular classes of antihypertensive agents?

COINDICATIONS	AGENTS
Atrial tachycardia and fibrillation	β-Blockers, verapamil, diltiazem
Diabetes mellitus (with nephropathy)	
Type 1	ACE inhibitors*
Type 2	Angiotensin II receptor blockers
Heart failure (systolic dysfunction)	ACE inhibitors* and diuretics
Myocardial infarction/coronary artery disease	β-Blockers
Prostatism	α_1-Antagonists
Renal insufficiency (causing renal artery stenosis)	ACE inhibitors*

* In patients for whom ACE inhibitors are indicated but who develop cough, angiotensin II receptor blockers can be used.

11. List some common comorbid conditions adversely affected by certain antihypertensives.

COMORBID CONDITION	ANTIHYPERTENSIVE
Asthma (bronchospasm)	β-Blockers
Gout	Diuretics
Heart block	β-Blockers, verapamil, diltiazem
Heart failure (systolic dysfunction)	Verapamil, diltiazem

12. How should the medication be prescribed initially?

Begin with moderate doses of medication, then follow up in 1- to 2-month intervals, adjusting upward as necessary until goal BP is reached. Rapid reduction of BP can precipitate target organ ischemia and should be avoided. Educate the patient about possible major adverse effects, and encourage the patient to contact you if he or she experiences severe or unremitting side effects.

13. What should be included in the follow-up visits?
- Careful measurement of BP, including orthostatic determinations in elderly patients
- Assessment of possible side effects (e.g, light-headedness, sexual dysfunction, edema)
- Measurement of blood urea nitrogen, serum creatinine, and electrolytes if the adjusted medication is an ACE inhibitor, angiotensin II receptor antagonist, or diuretic

14. Which questions should be asked to assess patient adherence to medication and lifestyle modification?
1. Is the patient taking the medication as prescribed? Can the patient afford and obtain the medication?

2. Is the patient experiencing any side effects? Assure the patient that you will work with them to minimize these or replace the medication with a better-tolerated substitute.

15. Is it preferable to maximize the dose of a single agent to achieve goal BP or to add another agent?
If the patient's BP responds to a medication and it is well tolerated, the next step is to increase the dose if necessary. If there is no response or the patient experiences undesirable side effects, it is appropriate either to switch to another agent or to add another agent if the initial medication is indicated for reasons other than BP (e.g., if the patient is diabetic and an ACE inhibitor is not having much effect, a diuretic can be added). A medication can be maximized as long as it is effective and tolerated until goal BP is reached.

16. Discuss which agents work best together.
Thiazide diuretics potentiate the effects of **ACE inhibitors** and work well with **β-blockers** and **calcium channel blockers**. They are especially useful in patients who have evidence of volume overload or have refractory hypertension. For patients with significant renal insufficiency (i.e., creatinine clearance < 30 mL/min), a **loop diuretic** should be used in place of a thiazide when diuretics are required to control BP.

α_1-**Antagonists** are useful adjuncts to any of the aforementioned agents except for the dihydropyridine calcium channel blockers (felodipine, nifedipine, amlodipine). Both classes can cause orthostasis and edema.

For patients who remain refractory despite attempts to treat with the aforementioned agents, consider the use of the **adrenergic antagonists**, reserpine (in low doses) or clonidine. Direct **vasodilators**, such as hydralazine and minoxidil, are effective but can cause edema and tachycardia. Diuretics and adrenergic antagonists are usually required in the antihypertensive regimen.

CONTROVERSIES

17. What medications have been proved to reduce overall cardiovascular morbidity and mortality?

Thiazide diuretics and **β-blockers** were the primary agents used in the initial randomized trials that ultimately proved that lowering BP in hypertensive patients reduced the risk of stroke, myocardial infarction, and overall cardiovascular mortality, and they are recommended as **first-line therapy** for hypertension.

Several trials have compared **angiotensin-converting enzyme (ACE) inhibitors** and **calcium channel blockers** with the older agents with regard to their impact on outcomes. To date, there is accumulating evidence that ACE inhibitors are effective, especially in high-risk patients such as diabetics. Although data also suggest that calcium channel blockers reduce cardiovascular morbidity and mortality, there is continuing controversy as to whether they are equally effective compared with ACE inhibitors as first-line agents.

18. Which antihypertensive medications are the best first-line choices?

Thiazide diuretics and **β-blockers** are recommended because there is ample evidence that they reduce cardiovascular morbidity and mortality, they are inexpensive, they can be taken once daily, and they are generally well tolerated. Evidence is accumulating, however, that **ACE inhibitors** reduce cardiovascular morbidity, renal morbidity, and overall mortality. They are well tolerated, relatively inexpensive, and can be taken once daily. Completion of several large comparative trials in the near future should clarify whether certain classes of antihypertensive agents exert a beneficial effect on cardiovascular morbidity and mortality compared with others.

BIBLIOGRAPHY

1. Blood Pressure Lowering Treatment Trialist's Collaboration: Effects of ACE inhibitors, calcium antagonists, and other BP-lowering drugs: Results of prospectively designed overviews of randomised trials. Lancet 356:1955–1964, 2000.
2. Jiang H, Whelton PK: Selection of initial antihypertensive drug therapy. Lancet 356:1942–1943, 2000.
3. Joint National Committee on Prevention, Detection, Evaluation, and Treatment of High Blood Pressure: The Sixth Report of the Joint National Committee on Prevention, Detection, Evaluation, and Treatment of High Blood Pressure. Arch Intern Med 157:2413–2445, 1997.
4. Pahor M, Psaty BM, Alderman MH, et al: Health outcomes associated with calcium antagonists compared with other first-line antihypertensive therapies: A meta-analysis of randomized controlled trials. Lancet 356:1949—1954, 2000.
5. Weir MR: Are drugs that block the renin-angiotensin system effective and safe in patients with renal insufficiency? Am J Hypertens 12:195S–203S, 1999.

INDEX